Group
Techniques
SECOND EDITION

D0197709

Group
Techniques
SECOND EDITION

Gerald Corey
California State University, Fullerton

Marianne Schneider Corey
Private Practice

Patrick Callanan
Private Practice

J. Michael Russell
California State University, Fullerton

Brooks/Cole Publishing Company
Pacific Grove, California

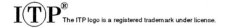

The ITP logo is a registered trademark under license.

Brooks/Cole Publishing Company
A Division of International Thomson Publishing Inc.

© 1992, 1988, 1982 by Brooks/Cole Publishing Co.
All rights reserved. No part of this book may be reproduced,
stored in a retrieval system, or transcribed, in any form or
by any means—electronic, mechanical, photocopying, recording,
or otherwise—without the prior written permission of the
publisher, Brooks/Cole Publishing Company, Pacific Grove,
California 93950.

Printed in the United States of America

10   9   8   7

Library of Congress Cataloging-in-Publication Data

Group techniques / Gerald Corey . . . [et al.]. — 2nd ed.
    p.   cm.
  Includes bibliographical references and index.
  ISBN 0-534-16248-7 :
  1. Group relations training.   I. Corey, Gerald.
HM134.G748   1991
302'.14—dc20   91-10852
                                                 CIP

Sponsoring Editor: *Claire Verduin*
Editorial Associate: *Gay C. Bond*
Production Editor: *Fiorella Ljunggren*
Manuscript Editor: *William Waller*
Permissions Editor: *Carline Haga*
Interior Design: *Vernon T. Boes*
Cover Design: *E. Kelly Shoemaker*
Typesetting: *Bookends Typesetting*
Printing and Binding: *Malloy Lithographing, Inc.*

Our book is dedicated to
the people who have been members in our groups,
especially those in our residential workshops,
who gave us the opportunity to learn more.

ABOUT THE AUTHORS

Gerald Corey is a professor of human services and counseling at California State University at Fullerton and was the coordinator of the university's Human Services Program from 1983 to 1991. A licensed psychologist, he received his doctorate in counseling from the University of Southern California. He is a Diplomate in Counseling Psychology, American Board of Professional Psychology; is registered as a National Health Service Provider in Psychology; is a National Certified Counselor; and is a licensed marriage, child, and family counselor. He is a Fellow of the American Psychological 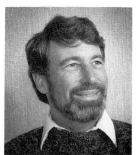 Association (Counseling Psychology) and a Fellow of the Association for Specialists in Group Work.

Each semester Jerry teaches courses in group counseling, group process, theory and practice of counseling, and professional ethics. With his colleagues, he has conducted workshops in the United States, Mexico, China, and Europe, with a special focus on training in group counseling, and he is often a guest lecturer at various universities. Along with the co-authors, each summer he offers weeklong residential personal-growth workshops in Idyllwild, California.

Jerry was the recipient of the 1991 Outstanding Professor of the Year Award from California State University at Fullerton; the 1988 Award for Contributions and Support of Human Service Education from the National Organization for Human Service Education; the 1986 Award in the Field of Professional Ethics from the Association for Religious and Value Issues in Counseling; the 1984 Distinguished Service Award in the Field of Group Work from the Association for Specialists in Group Work; and the 1984 Distinguished Faculty Member Award from the School of Human Development and Community Service of California State University at Fullerton.

The recent books he has authored or co-authored (all published by Brooks/Cole Publishing Company) are:

- *Groups: Process and Practice,* Fourth Edition (1992)
- *Case Approach to Counseling and Psychotherapy,* Third Edition (1991)
- *Theory and Practice of Counseling and Psychotherapy,* Fourth Edition (and *Manual*) (1991)
- *I Never Knew I Had a Choice,* Fourth Edition (1990)
- *Theory and Practice of Group Counseling,* Third Edition (and *Manual*) (1990)
- *Becoming a Helper* (1989)
- *Issues and Ethics in the Helping Professions,* Third Edition (1988)

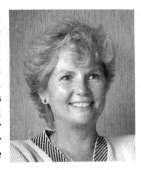

Marianne Schneider Corey is a licensed marriage and family therapist in Idyllwild, California, and is a National Certified Counselor. She received her master's degree in marriage, family, and child counseling from Chapman College. She is a Fellow of the Association for Specialists in Group Work, a clinical member of the American Association for Marriage and Family Therapy and holds membership in the California Association of Marriage and Family Therapists, the American Association for Counseling and Development, the Association for Religious and Value Issues in Counseling, and the National Organization for Human Service Education.

Marianne's professional interests include counseling individuals and couples, as well as leading therapeutic groups and training groups for mental-health professionals. She also trains and supervises student leaders in a group-counseling class and co-leads weeklong residential growth groups at California State University at Fullerton. With her colleagues, she has conducted professional workshops in the United States, Mexico, China, and Europe. She received an Award for Contributions to the Field of Professional Ethics from the Association for Religious and Value Issues in Counseling in 1986.

Marianne has co-authored the following books (all published by Brooks/Cole Publishing Company):

- *Groups: Process and Practice,* Fourth Edition (1992)
- *I Never Knew I Had a Choice,* Fourth Edition (1990)
- *Becoming a Helper* (1989)
- *Issues and Ethics in the Helping Professions,* Third Edition (1988)

She has also co-authored several articles published in the *Journal for Specialists in Group Work,* the most recent of which is "Role of Group Leader's Values in Group Counseling" (May 1990), with Patrick Callanan and Gerald Corey.

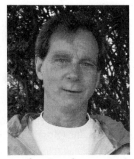

Patrick Callanan is a licensed marriage and family therapist in private practice in Santa Ana, California, and is a National Certified Counselor. He received his master's degree in professional psychology from United States International University.

Patrick is on the part-time faculty of the Human Services Program at California State University at Fullerton, where he regularly teaches an internship course, assists in training and supervising group leaders, and co-leads weeklong residential growth groups. He is a consultant for mental-health practitioners, and he also presents workshops and training groups at conventions and for professional organizations. He is a member of the California Association of Marriage and Family Therapists, the Association for Specialists in Group Work, and the American Association for Counseling and Development. He received an Award for Contributions to the Field of Professional Ethics from the Association for Religious and Value Issues in Counseling in 1986.

Patrick has co-authored several articles published in the *Journal for Specialists in Group Work,* including "Role of Group Leader's Values in Group Counseling" (May 1990), with Marianne and Gerald Corey. He has also co-authored, with Marianne and Gerald Corey, the following book (published by Brooks/Cole Publishing Company):

* *Issues and Ethics in the Helping Professions,* Third Edition (1988)

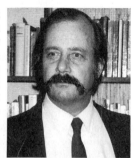

J. Michael Russell is professor of philosophy and human services at California State University at Fullerton, a psychoanalyst in private practice, and a core faculty member of the Newport Psychoanalytic Institute, where he teaches courses on psychoanalysis and is chair of the training committee. He has been leading workshops and teaching courses in personal growth since 1971, when he obtained his doctorate in philosophy from the University of California at Santa Barbara. His philosophical interest in self-deception broadened into courses he teaches in philosophical assumptions of psychotherapy, existentialism and phenomenology, theories and techniques of counseling, case analysis, and group leadership and into workshops he conducts in leadership training. He became a National Certified Counselor in 1984, a registered Research Psychoanalyst in 1985, and a Graduate Psychoanalyst in 1988. He is a member of several professional organizations, including the American Association for Counseling and Development, the Association for Specialists in Group Work, the Society for Phenomenology and Existential Philosophy, and the American Philosophical Association. His publications include, among others, the following articles:

* "The Human Services Program at California State University, Fullerton" (with Corey, Coley, Ramirez, and Wright), in *Journal of Counseling and Human Services* (May 1986)
* "Desires Don't Cause Actions," in *Journal of Mind and Behavior* (Winter 1984)
* "Ethical Considerations in Using Group Techniques" (with Corey, Corey, and Callanan), in *Journal for Specialists in Group Work* (September 1982)
* "Reflection and Self-Deception," in *Journal for Research in Phenomenology* (1981, Volume II)
* "A Report of a Weeklong Residential Workshop for Personal Growth" (with Corey, Corey, and Callanan), in *Journal for Specialists in Group Work* (November 1980)
* "How to Think about Thinking: A Preliminary Map," in *Journal of Mind and Behavior* (Spring 1980)

PREFACE

Since the four of us began working together in 1972, we have been involved in almost every aspect of group work as members, leaders, teachers, and workshop conductors. In the course of this long involvement we have found ourselves continually faced with questions about techniques in groups—their place, their usefulness, their abuse. In many of our training workshops we have observed beginning leaders flounder in their use of techniques. In professional workshops we have fielded questions implying that there is or should be a scientific body of techniques available to the practitioner to cover every eventuality in a group.

Our primary assumption in this book is that techniques are never the main course in group work. This assumption has many implications. It puts the focus on the members and the leader and on the quality of the interactions between them. Techniques are means, not ends; they are not to be hidden behind and are not to be forced on the client; they should be used to increase knowledge and awareness. They are fundamentally at the service of the client, not the therapist.

To avoid having the techniques described in this book used as the primary focus of group work, we do not attempt to provide an exhaustive catalog of techniques and exercises. Our purpose is not to outline all possible techniques for every possible population but to teach leaders how to develop and use techniques in group work. You can best use this book by reading a chapter, putting the book down, and then asking yourself what relevance the techniques described have for you in your situation and how they might be applied. We hope you will not borrow our techniques verbatim and use them without consideration for the members of your groups and their unique relationships with you and with one another.

In addition, we expect that this book will stimulate your interest in the broad field of working with people in groups and in the philosophical and ethical dimensions of what you do. Such an interest could lead you to think about theories of therapy, to further your own therapy, to engage in exchanges of ideas rather than being professionally isolated, and to participate in professional workshops. It could also lead you to an interest in supervision, whether in the formal sense of learning or in the informal sense of working with a respected colleague. If this book motivates you to broaden your interest to encompass the whole field of counseling and therapy, we believe that interest will help to diminish the abuse of techniques.

We sought to write this book in a style that fits our personal perspective and our way of leading groups. We have not included references to other authors within the body of the text, except for the Association for Specialists in Group Work (ASGW). This is the main professional organization for those interested in group work. The ASGW has developed ethical guidelines for group practice and also training standards for group workers. We make reference to these ethical guidelines when they are relevant to the issues being discussed. We also provide a selected bibliography at the end of the book to further your thinking about group work. Even though we do not make references to other sources, let us add that the techniques we discuss did not arise in a vacuum. In addition to being direct responses to problems presented by participants in groups we have led, the techniques in this book bear the stamp of our own therapists, of leaders of groups and workshops in which we have been members, and of a great many writers with various theoretical orientations.

This book is for students and practitioners in any human-services field, from counseling psychology to social work, where the group is an accepted modality. In the classroom it can be a valuable auxiliary text in basic group courses and in a practicum in group work. The techniques described in this book are most appropriately used when counseling groups with an open-ended agenda. In practice the book can be used to stimulate thinking and creativity in one's approach to group work, and it can be used in conjunction with supervision. Intended readers include psychiatric nurses, social workers, psychologists, ministers, marriage and family therapists, teachers, and mental-health professionals and paraprofessionals who lead groups.

In this second edition of *Group Techniques* we have fine-tuned the various techniques. We have given increased attention to clients' cultural diversity in Chapter 1 and have also included a discussion of cultural issues as a factor in the use of group techniques. In Chapter 2, we have provided expanded coverage of ethics as it applies to group techniques.

This edition contains more specific examples for each of the stages of a group, and expanded coverage of the guidelines and suggestions for group members. We have also included contrasting descriptions of time-limited and long-term groups and how to set them up. The initial stage and the transition stage now cover two chapters, and the material in Chapters 3, 4, and 5 has been rearranged to flow more smoothly. In this revision our aim has been to focus on practical applications. Although we take an eclectic stance and avoid a single theoretical bias, we emphasize throughout that theory must guide a practitioner's interventions. We hope that the tone and spirit of this book will encourage group leaders to develop their own therapeutic styles. At the same time, we recommend necessary cautions, both procedural and ethical, as group leaders design and implement various techniques.

We would like to thank Peg Carroll of Fairfield University, Barbara Herlihy of the University of Houston at Clear Lake, and David Zimpfer of Kent State University, who read the revised manuscript and provided us with constructive suggestions. We also appreciate Katie Dutro's contribution as a student reviewer and as an indexer and Debbie DeBue's assistance in typing the manuscript.

We wish to express our appreciation to the dedicated members of the Brooks/Cole team—Fiorella Ljunggren, production services manager, and Claire Verduin, managing editor and psychology editor—for their interest in the revision process and for their helpful perspectives. We are especially indebted to William Waller, the manuscript editor, whose editorial skills helped us produce a clear and readable book.

Gerald Corey
Marianne Schneider Corey
Patrick Callanan
J. Michael Russell

CONTENTS

Group
Techniques
SECOND EDITION

The Role of Techniques

At the outset, we want to specify what we mean by the word *technique.* The definition is not as simple as it may sound. Virtually anything a group leader does could be viewed as a technique, including being silent, suggesting a new behavior, inviting a client to explore a conflict, maintaining eye contact, arranging seating, offering reactions to members, and presenting interpretations. To be more precise, however, we generally use the term *technique* to refer to a leader's explicit and directive request of a member for the purpose of focusing on material, augmenting or exaggerating affect, practicing behavior, or solidifying insight. This definition includes the following procedures: conducting initial interviews, in which members are asked to focus on their reasons for wanting to join a group; asking a nonproductive group to clarify the direction it wants to take; asking a member to role-play a specific situation; asking a member to practice a behavior; encouraging a person to repeat certain words or to complete a sentence; helping members summarize what they have learned from a group session; challenging a member's belief system; and working with the cognitions that influence a member's behavior. We also consider as techniques those procedures aimed at helping group leaders get a sense of the direction they might pursue with a group.

Avoiding the Misuse of Techniques

Misconceptions about the use of techniques abound. When we give workshops on groups, participants sometimes ask us to suggest techniques for working with specific clients. The implication seems to be that to lead a group effectively, one should have the "right" technical tools to employ at the "right" moment. Perhaps for some models of group counseling, such as behavior modification, specific methods are appropriate to achieve well-defined behavioral outcomes. In many types of groups, however, the techniques that are most useful grow out of the work of the participants and are tailored to the situations that evolve in a particular session.

Given our assumption that techniques are means and not ends, we naturally have some concerns about how this book will be used: Will the book contribute to the problem of group leaders' overemphasizing techniques? Will readers memorize specific devices and use them insensitively, rather than treating the book as a means to deepen their own therapeutic inventiveness and judgment? In both cases, of course, we hope not. We would like instead to challenge leaders to use their creativity and to take risks in inventing techniques spontaneously.

It is impossible to predict what the exact nature of a group will be. Thus, a recipe-book approach to therapeutic techniques, while providing opportunities to try different procedures, surely does not replace the main function of a group leader. Many an excellent cook—and this would be our recommendation for the therapist—creates a different dish each time. Even though working from a basic recipe, one has to follow one's taste, use foods available at the market that day, and trust one's own sensitivity.

Paying attention to the obvious. It is our assumption that techniques can deepen feelings that are already present and that they should preferably grow out of what is already taking place. When a person says "I'm feeling lonely," for example, it is appropriate to introduce a technique to help move this feeling further. For this reason, we generally prefer to include the members in the selection of group themes rather than to select a theme arbitrarily. This is not a hard-and-fast rule; many group practitioners work effectively with preselected techniques, exercises, and themes. Indeed, for certain populations, this approach is indicated. Many short-term structured groups make use of topics and exercises as ways to help members learn. Thus, techniques are employed to help members accomplish their personal goals within the framework of the group's basic purpose.

In the groups we lead, we tend to use techniques to initiate material at the beginning of a group and often use them to summarize material at the end. Instead of using techniques to "make something happen," we generally use them for elaborating on what is already happening. We tend to avoid having too rigid an agenda for the group process; instead, we emphasize the value of letting members lead the way. We find that it is best to follow the energy and the clues provided by the members, rather than being overly directive.

Many groups have moments of stagnation or resistance. It is easy in these situations—and often unwise—to hasten to employ a technique to get things moving rather than to pay attention to the important material being presented. Instead, it can be therapeutically useful to teach the members how to assess what is occurring in the group process and how to mobilize the group's energy. By looking around the room, for example, you may notice that members show signs of being disengaged; they appear bored, they are fidgeting, or they are falling asleep. We think the best technique at such times is to ask the members about their sense of what's happening. You might say: "I'm willing to work hard to help you get what you came for. I'm also aware that many of you do not seem interested. Few of you are speaking up, there is a good deal of fidgeting, people are not responding to one another, and I feel as though I'm doing most of the work. I'd like to hear from each of you what is happening with you now." You can then share your feelings at the moment, or you can save them until the members have expressed what they are feeling. What should be avoided is trying technique after technique to stimulate movement in a situation such as this. We prefer to deal with what is actually occurring within the group by describing without judgment the behavior we are observing and by encouraging the members to decide what they want to do about their level of involvement in the group.

In addition, when considering whether to introduce a technique, you should take into account the stage of the group's development. For instance, you can expect trust to be an issue at the initial stage of a group. A group may be somewhat silent and cautious at this point in its existence. To introduce a technique to get things moving is to ignore the obvious and to impose a dynamic that is either premature for the group or alien to its character.

Doing so tends to interfere with the group's natural development. By introducing a technique that stresses and clarifies what is happening, you augment the process rather than intrude on it.

Maintaining flexibility. As leaders of groups, we encourage you to develop flexibility about which material to work with, rather than being rigid about where a technique is supposed to go. It is important that you be ready to flow wherever the material may lead. Thus, be prepared to abandon a technique that seems to lead nowhere or to modify it as needed. We once witnessed a therapist demonstrating work with an angry woman. He kept urging her to hit a pillow with her hands, apparently failing to notice or being too rigid to adjust to the fact that she was already twisting it. It would have been more appropriate to work with the material she was presenting. To take a different illustration, a leader may determine that a client needs to pursue an issue with her father. The leader may introduce a technique designed to accentuate her sadness and yet should be ready to work with her showing anger instead. In a group-therapy session we supervised, a violent patient kept reiterating that he was "different." The leader insisted on this client's dealing with his violent feelings rather than exploring his more pressing concern about being different. Either theme could have been worked with, but it seemed to us that the session did not progress as much as it might have because of the therapist's idea of the direction the client should be taking. By being open to members' needs at the moment, the group leader can assess what techniques to draw on in helping them work on salient themes that they determine.

Although it is possible to make mistakes because of insensitivity to promising and pressing material, we would not want leaders to become too anxious about pursuing the "right" or the "most pressing" material. There is often no single "right" way to proceed. If we become too focused on doing exactly the right thing at the right time, we are likely to stifle our creativity and miss important clues that participants give us. Often, several directions are equally worth pursuing. When we are asked why we chose one direction rather than another in a given situation, we frequently feel that we could also have taken the work in a different direction. Here our own interests and level of energy come into play.

The Therapeutic Relationship

Much of clients' opportunity for significant change is based on their relationship with the group leader. Just as many of the behaviors we label maladaptive had their origins in faulty early relationships, new and more appropriate behaviors can be cemented through the new relationship with the leader. If this relationship is inauthentic, superficial, or otherwise impoverished, we doubt that clients will make significant strides in making desired changes. Changes must be tried out, and the therapeutic relationship provides this testing ground. Let's look at two issues in the use of techniques that illustrate the significance of the therapeutic relationship—timing and avoiding self-deception.

Timing the use of techniques.   A critical skill in group work is using techniques with consideration for whether clients are prepared to give up their defenses. To push beyond clients' readiness to move is to violate their integrity. To assault defenses without consideration for their importance in maintaining equilibrium is to expose clients to possible psychological damage. No technique will provide you with information on how ready clients are to give up their defenses. You need intelligence, wisdom, and, above all, a concerned attentiveness to your relationship with your clients. This relationship provides them with the hold on reality they need to move away from nonproductive and excessively defensive conduct. As group members learn to trust and believe in you, they are likely to move toward personal freedom. In the absence of such a relationship, they are being asked to trust techniques without any sign of your concern for them. Clients in that position do well to resist. The therapist who pays attention to the leader/client relationship develops a sixth sense that makes it possible to gauge the course of therapy and to judge the optimum time for gently pushing clients into areas previously avoided. This skill is above and beyond technique. To some degree it is a part of the therapist's makeup, but it can be refined through training and supervision.

Avoiding self-deception in using techniques.   Techniques can be powerful sources for emotional release and can generate tremendous energy in the therapeutic group. But they can easily mask the relationship between the leader and the members. When the storm has subsided, any insights gained can be easily dismissed by clients as having been brought about by something foreign to their own resources: the power of a special environment or the magic of the leader's technical skills. At the other extreme, because of the impact of a cathartic moment, clients can cling to the false belief that the issue has now been worked on and is finished. Catharsis can be exciting, and yet it can feed a false sense of productivity. The leader who is too hungry to produce a heavy emotional session may use techniques to generate the appearance of movement without being sensitive to the need to work the material through and to gain some comprehension of its meaning and implications.

Choosing Techniques for Various Types of Groups

The type of group that you lead will determine to a large degree the appropriateness of various techniques. Some techniques may be ideally suited for a therapy group or a counseling group, yet they may not be appropriate for certain groups with an educational focus. The majority of the techniques that we describe in this book work best in counseling groups and therapy groups. Some of the techniques that we describe in the chapters on the transition and working stages, for example, would not be suitable for a short-term structured group with children. However, our purpose is not to present techniques with the idea that you will copy them. Instead, we aim to provide you with many examples of techniques that we have used with our therapeutic groups in the hope that you will think about ways to create a range of your own techniques suited to your particular population and your specific groups.

In designing your groups, you will certainly need to focus clearly on the basic goal you hope to attain. The time structure, the setting, the techniques you employ, the candidates you accept for the group, and your role as leader are all largely determined by the type of group you are designing. With respect to the role that techniques will play in your group, it is of central importance to consider how they can be used in the service of clients. In certain task groups, you may want to employ structured exercises and make use of a clear agenda that will guide your group sessions. If you are conducting a guidance or psychoeducational group for adolescents in a school, you may rule out certain techniques that are designed to bring about an exploration of intense emotions. In creating and using techniques, therefore, you will always want to keep clearly in mind the primary purpose of your group. Techniques will be tools to help you and your members accomplish the group's specific aims.

In addition to a range of suggestions about recruiting, screening, informing, and preparing group members (see Chapter 3), we recommend a generic technique for virtually all groups. This consists of some form of invitation for members to declare *their* perception of the group, what they want from it, or something that will involve them in formulating the group's direction. Specific suggestions for these "check-ins" will be found throughout the book. We routinely ask group members at the outset of a workshop, a group course, or a session of an ongoing group to say something about what particular hopes, expectations, fantasies, and fears they are bringing with them to the group.

In any given situation in a group, several different techniques can often be used, and each may be equally beneficial to a client. What basis does a leader have for choosing one technique rather than another? Leaders do well to consider factors such as their theoretical orientation, the population that makes up the group, the personality of the individual member and the group leader, and the client's cultural context.

Theory as a basis. The theoretical persuasion of the group leader often dictates the selection of a technique. For example, free association by clients with minimal intrusion from the leader usually leads to regression and a re-experiencing of earlier memories. Asking clients to pay attention to what they are thinking and feeling as others are working tends to focus a person on the here and now. Techniques of reinforcement for behavior direct attention away from intrapersonal dynamics. Thus, the choice of techniques depends to some extent on the theoretical framework of the therapist.

Ideally, you will be open to devising techniques that tap the thinking, feeling, and behaving dimensions of human experience. Each of the theoretical frameworks has a good deal to offer in providing strategies for creative work. At times, members need to experience their feelings more deeply. At other times, they can benefit from exploring their beliefs and assumptions, some of which may be self-limiting. Still, there is a time when members need to develop an action plan for translating their insights into new behaviors. The same person can profit from a different focus at various stages in his or her work.

Client population as a basis.   A sensitivity to the population with whom you are dealing should be manifest in the techniques you choose. One cannot use the same techniques with a group of hospital patients with organic brain syndrome that one would use with clients in a growth group. Similarly, techniques that tend to bring strong emotions to the surface need to be used cautiously with a group for the criminally insane. Techniques used for group-therapy clients may be inappropriate for professionals such as nurses or teachers in a group for developing interpersonal skills. There is an almost limitless variety of groups, and a leader needs to ask constantly: "Is this technique suitable for this group of people? Is it the best available technique for this population in this situation?"

Client personality as a basis.   A technique should also be chosen with the personality of the individual client in mind. If it does not fit, it does not facilitate the genuine meeting of human beings. Imagine asking a reserved, middle-aged, upper-class woman to use four-letter words as an expression of her anger. Although the therapist may feel it valuable for her to express anger, it is equally important to respect her sensitivity to such language. There must be a congruence of the technique, the person introducing it, and the person for whom it is intended.

Adapting group techniques to the client's cultural context.   In choosing techniques, it is essential to consider the ways in which the client's cultural background influences his or her personality and values. Some clients, because of their cultural conditioning, are averse to expressing emotions openly or to talking freely about problems within their family. If a technique goes against the grain of a member's personality, it will probably result in alienating the client from the group. The key is to present techniques in a way that respects the uniqueness of an individual's personal and cultural context.

If you expect to lead groups with culturally diverse populations, it will be essential that you discover ways to modify your strategies to meet their needs. Perhaps your genuine respect for the differences among members in your groups and your willingness to learn from them will be the most important foundation on which to build a bridge between yourself and them. It is particularly critical to monitor your own behavior so that you will avoid making rigid and stereotyped generalizations about individuals within a particular social or cultural group.

It is a mistake to assume that a common set of techniques can be applied equally to all people in groups irrespective of their cultural background. In leading groups, it is essential to acquire both the sensitivity and the knowledge to modify various techniques to fit the client's background. According to the Association for Specialists in Group Work (ASGW), it is the responsibility of leaders to inform potential members before they join of the values that will guide group interaction.* For instance, these values may include staying in the here and now, expressing feelings, asking for what one wants, being direct and honest, sharing personal material with others, making oneself known to others, learning how to trust, improving interpersonal communication, learning to take the initiative, dealing with conflict, being willing to confront others, and deciding for oneself. Because of their cultural background and the values they hold, certain clients may have difficulty with techniques and group procedures that reflect some of these values. Certain members may have difficulty being direct, because their culture has reinforced the norm of indirectness. Other clients may experience trouble in putting themselves in the central place or in taking up group time, largely because they have learned from their culture that to do so is rude and insensitive. Some members will not be comfortable in making decisions for themselves, because their culture has taught them to follow traditional standards or authorities outside of themselves. Although some group techniques are designed to assist members in more freely expressing their feelings, certain members will find this offensive. They may have been taught that it is good to keep their feelings to themselves and that it is improper to display emotional reactions publicly.

The ASGW guidelines specify that "group counselors are aware of their own values and assumptions and how they apply in a multicultural context." A related guideline cautions leaders about the dangers of stereotyping members because of such factors as their age, gender, or cultural background:

> Group counselors take steps to increase their awareness of ways that their personal reactions to members might inhibit the group process and they monitor their countertransference. Through an awareness of the impact of stereotyping and discrimination (i.e., biases based on age, disability, ethnicity, gender, race, religion, or sexual preference), group counselors guard the individual rights and personal dignity of all group members.

Cultural diversity affects the issues that members bring to a group and the ways in which they might be either ready or reluctant to explore these issues. Group leaders would do well to sensitize themselves to the clues that

*From *Ethical Guidelines for Group Counselors,* by the Association for Specialists in Group Work. Copyright 1989 by the American Association for Counseling and Development. This and all other quotations from the same source are reprinted by permission. Consult the Appendix for a copy of these guidelines.

members often give indicating that they would like to talk about some aspect of how their culture is affecting their participation in the group.

It is possible to create techniques that give members an opportunity to talk about certain aspects of their culture. Several examples come to mind. Ramon had a difficult time with a female co-leader who tended to be very direct and say exactly what was on her mind. His culture had conditioned him to use more indirect ways of communicating. Ramon had particular difficulty with a woman speaking her mind with such candor, for in his culture women were supposed to be quiet and unassertive, and it was not appropriate for a woman to confront a man. He let the leader know that he did want to talk about this situation, for he also experienced problems with assertive women outside the group. Another member, Rosalie, wanted an opportunity to let others in the group know that she had a hard time in letting others take care of her. Her culture had reinforced her behavior of taking care of all her brothers and sisters, but it had not reinforced her for asking for others to nurture her. This is one reason that she had such difficulty in letting others in the group give to her and why she devoted so much energy to taking care of everyone else in the group who expressed pain. Both Ramon and Rosalie felt that they were better understood after they had had a chance to let others know what their culture had taught them and how these lessons were affecting their behavior in the group. After they felt that others understood their cultural frame of reference, it was possible to introduce techniques that would accentuate selected cultural themes and help these members decide in what ways they might want to modify some of their behavior. Ramon experimented with being a bit more direct and telling the female co-leader how she affected him; Rosalie tried a new behavior when she told others in the group one way in which she could let each of them care for her.

We highlight cultural material as it emerges in a group session by providing individuals with an invitation to identify relevant dimensions of their culture. We might suggest any of the following:

- "Tell us something about your culture and how you think it may influence your participation in this group."
- "If you think many members of this group might have a certain cultural perspective different from your own, would you pick out some people here and tell each of them about some of the things that you are likely to see differently?"
- "Could you pretend for a moment that you're back home among members of your ethnic group? Try to explain to them what this group is all about. What would you say?"
- (To a specific member): "I'm aware that many of us in this group are from a culture that is different from yours. Would you be interested in some of us expressing some of our assumptions or stereotypes about your culture? You can then react to what you hear, which could be a means for us to find out more from you about how we could reconsider some of our conclusions."

The point of techniques of this kind is to bring certain cultural material to the surface so that potential conflicts or misunderstandings can be dealt with openly. If these themes remain latent, unspoken thoughts and unexpressed reactions are likely to interfere with the development of cohesion. Although members do share in universal human concerns, the members are also different from one another. A group is an ideal place for people to learn how to understand, appreciate, and respect their cultural differences at the same time as they discover ways in which they are bonded by common denominators.

Introducing Techniques

Learn to pay attention to how you introduce techniques. To what extent do you explain them? How do you ask members to participate in them? How do you work with members who are reluctant to follow your suggestions?

Explaining techniques.   You can't always explain to a client in detail what the proposed technique is, the rationale for its use, and the desired outcome. To do so may render the technique useless. For instance, a lengthy explanation may interrupt the flow of the material. Or an explanation that specifies an anticipated emotion—"You'll probably experience a lot of pain and cry if you do this"—may set the client up to artificially display that feeling or to talk about it. In our groups we also do not usually try to explain the outcome, exactly because we ourselves are not always sure what may develop. For example, a woman says she feels she may be too critical, and so we later introduce an exercise that encourages her to be critical, based on our hunch that being critical is indeed a part of her. Although we suspect the outcome, we leave it to the process to prove whether our hunch is correct. We do not mean to imply that everything about techniques has to be mysterious. Part of the preparation of group members should include discussion about techniques and how they serve the purpose of a group. In our groups we discuss the limitations we place on ourselves in how far we are willing to go in the use of techniques. We sometimes mention the experiences we have had with techniques in our personal therapy. This kind of explanation does little to make techniques ineffective and may greatly lessen clients' fears of them.

Inviting members to participate.   It is our practice to invite group members to go along with a technique and to proceed only when we sense that we have their permission. We tend to use such phrases as these: "Are you willing to take this further?" "Are you willing to try this?" "I have something in mind that might help you understand better what you are saying. Let me tell you what it is, and see whether you are willing to go along with it." Especially when we are working with clients with a cultural background different from ours, we take an invitational stance that both offers respect and encourages clients to challenge their values and behaviors. If we are working with Brian, a client who is ethnically different from us, we make room for the fact that his differences might partially account for behavior in the group that could be perceived as "resistance." For example, he may be very quiet yet observant in the group, and he may seek advice from us about what would be the right course for him to take in coping with his problems. We do not quickly assume that he is detached, resistant, and dependent. Instead, we pursue with him the possible meanings of certain of his behaviors. In doing so, we may learn that he is silent because he has learned that this is a sign of respect. His culture may have taught him not to put the focus of attention on himself. Also, his conditioning may prime him to seek direction from people he considers authorities. By respectfully gathering data about Brian with his help, we are in a better position to teach him ways to get what he needs from the group without violating his cultural norms.

Working with clients' reluctance. If group members say that they are not willing to participate in an exercise, we might ask "Are you willing to talk about why you're hesitating?" If the answer is still negative, we usually let it go, but we keep the incident in mind. If clients develop a style of declining invitations to work, we point it out to them and ask them if they are interested in doing anything about this pattern. We take this position on the basis that, on the one hand, clients should not be harassed or pushed into doing what they are unwilling to do but that, on the other hand, a group often needs to exert some pressure if many clients are to get work done.

Note that we ask our clients to talk about why they do not want to go along with a technique. This is a genuine request, and we do not automatically label their behavior resistance. Brian's case, which we just presented, is a good illustration of how we can work with what appears to be a member's reluctance to participate in a respectful, yet challenging, manner.

We think that a lot of "resistance" is justified caution on the part of the client. Most often members are willing to talk about their reluctance, and almost inevitably this discussion leads to important issues for the group, such as the trust or distrust felt toward certain members or perhaps toward the leader. Hence, at this point the sensitive leader abandons the technique, perhaps introducing a different technique appropriate for pursuing the theme of lack of trust. For example, the leader might now say: "I would like to be able to work with you, but I'm having trouble knowing how to proceed. You've indicated that you don't feel safe in here yet, and that perhaps explains your reluctance to go along with some of the exercises. I really hope that you're willing to talk about what it would take for you to feel more trusting in here. Would you be willing to say to each person in this group— myself included—something about each of us that makes it easy or difficult for you to feel trust?" This technique can lead to good outcomes for the group, increased cohesion, and willingness in the future to go along with suggested techniques.

The Leader as a Person

We want to emphasize the leader's involvement in moving the group forward. In this regard, the leader's character, personal qualities, and philosophy of life are more important than any technique for facilitating the group process. You, as a group leader, are more than the sum total of your skills. From this viewpoint, when you take from another source a technique that is not a reflection of your own character, you are introducing something that is alien to you. For instance, if you are a low-key person and you introduce a highly dramatic technique, chances are that the discrepancy will inhibit the group. You can, instead, use your unique personal qualities as a part of your therapeutic style. You may have a wit that can be used appropriately. Your playfulness can become an integral part of how you facilitate a group. Whatever personal dimension you draw from, it is critical to remember that in many ways the person who you are is your best therapeutic instrument.

Too often those who lead groups look for techniques for every possible occurrence. They overrely on techniques to pull themselves out of difficult situations, to get groups moving, or to keep them moving, and in doing so they become mechanical facilitators. This practice ignores the most powerful resource for reaching group members: the leader's personal reactions to the members and to what is going on in the group.

It is important that you acquire knowledge of how groups function, learn the necessary skills and techniques to implement your knowledge in actual group work, and do so in such a way that your techniques become an expression of your personal style and an extension of the unique person you are. We hope that you will take what we have to offer in these chapters and create your own variations—that you will develop a recipe that suits your taste. We are proposing an experimental attitude, and we encourage you to try out techniques and different ways of working in a group to gradually learn what works for you, as well as what does not.

How can you use techniques that are an extension of yourself as a person? We'd like to make some suggestions that will enhance your use of techniques and that will help you acquire a style that fits your personality.

Pay attention to yourself. A good place to begin is by monitoring your own experience in the group, including looking at the impact you have on the members. This process involves assessing your level of investment, your directness, your willingness to model what you expect of your members, and your willingness to be psychologically present for them. How great are your own energy and your own readiness to be responsive to the group? You will tune into the group more sensitively if you are in the habit of tuning into yourself. Indeed, one of the best ways to evaluate the energy of a group is to learn to assess your own energy as a barometer.

Learn to trust yourself. Learning to trust yourself is another essential part of the task of finding a style that suits your personality. If you do not trust your hunches, you may hold yourself back from even trying certain techniques. One way to develop this kind of trust is by being willing to follow your hunches and by trying variations of the techniques we describe. If a technique doesn't work, the consequences don't have to be horrible. Simply acknowledging that an exercise or a technique is not working is often the best way of pulling yourself out of a situation that could otherwise become worse. It is clearly not helpful to worry too much about making mistakes. If you aren't willing to make some mistakes, if you are bound by being sure before you act, you will miss many opportunities for action, and your clients will be deprived of opportunities as well. We admit that what we advocate takes courage. It takes a willingness to admit errors.

Model. Another way to be sure that your use of techniques reflects your personality is through modeling. Be aware of your thoughts and feelings as they surface within you in a group, and be willing to voice them. In so doing, you communicate to your group that it is acceptable to have and to show feelings and to express your thoughts. Through your own modeling, you open the way for members to express themselves. For example, if you are feeling blue and express this sadness, your resulting ability and willingness to be touched by others who are sad and to empathize with them can help them fully explore the experience and the meaning of their sadness. Your behavior can be a catalyst in assisting those members to explore rather than to cut off their feelings. If you are not afraid of emotional intensity and if you keep in contact with members as they share deep feelings, then other members are likely to face and deal with their struggles.

Modeling is not a technique to stir up feelings but an invitation to members to get in contact with their experience largely through your example. A potential danger is that you may end up expressing your personal concerns more often than any member of the group. If you become aware of doing so, you need to ask yourself: "Am I using the group for self-indulgent purposes? Am I at a point where personal counseling for myself is indicated?" Your self-disclosures should be relevant to what is going on in the group, and the time you take should not be at the members' expense. Your disclosures should facilitate self-exploration and interaction within the group rather than burdening the members with your personal issues.

In addition to encouraging members to express their feelings, you can also influence their behaviors through modeling. You can invite members to broaden their range of group behavior by demonstrating certain behaviors yourself. You can teach directness through your own directness. You can encourage members to give sensitive and honest feedback to others by doing so yourself. If you model nonjudgmental confrontation in a way that shows your concern for the person being challenged, your group members will learn how to confront one another in the same fashion. And through your openness, you invite members to share what they are experiencing.

Approaching group sessions with a sense of enthusiasm generates enthusiasm within the group. Your vitality and your being psychologically present for members are in themselves powerful modeling agents in getting groups to move. Your degree of aliveness and enthusiasm may be an index of the degree to which your groups are able to function in a vital way.

In summary, techniques have more impact if you are able to maintain a relationship with group members that is based on trust. Such trust is best created through the personal qualities that you project. In other words, techniques do not work in isolation from your personality and your relationship with members. You make a difference.

Concluding Comments

The key point of this chapter is that techniques are valuable and important but must be used with caution. Because of the immediate progress that techniques seem to promote, the therapist may draw on them rigidly and mechanically or may fail to explore material that they bring out. Techniques should be chosen in and for the situation; they are not to be memorized and then imposed on the group process. Our main concern in this book is not to equip you with an arsenal of group strategies but to encourage you to invent techniques that are extensions of yourself and your own sensitivities. We certainly are not urging you to memorize the techniques discussed in this book. Instead, you should use the book as a tool for improving your own ability to devise techniques and to think through the rationale for and the possible consequences of the techniques you invent.

Rather than going directly on to Chapter 2 now, you may find it useful to turn instead to Chapter 8, "In a Nutshell." The outline of key ideas and concepts in that chapter provides a good review of the material we have covered in this first chapter. Reading Chapter 8 at this time will provide you with an overview of the points that we will expand on in the remainder of the book and with a basis for understanding our philosophy and the way we lead groups.

Questions and Activities

At the end of each chapter we include a section of questions and activities. We hope you will use them to review the chapter and to clarify your own positions and integrate what you have read. Or you may prefer to spend your time thinking about issues we have not included. We list far more questions and activities than we think anyone will be interested in pursuing in depth. We encourage you to read all the questions and then select the ones that have the most interest and value for you, modifying them to match your own interests, client population, and situation. If you are using this book as a classroom text, many of the questions and activities listed can be adapted for small-group discussion, role playing, essay questions, and debates. The activities can be tried out in experiential groups.

As you review each chapter, you may have thoughts about how it could have been made clearer or more comprehensive. We hope that you will send us your reactions. You will find at the end of this book a form on which you can share your reactions with us. Mail it directly to us at Brooks/Cole Publishing Company, Pacific Grove, CA 93950-5098.

1. How would you define a technique? What is your view of the role that techniques should ideally play in the group process?
2. As a group leader, to what extent do you use techniques, and when do you think it is appropriate or inappropriate to do so? How does your use of techniques fit with your overall view of what a group is for?
3. We stated some of our concerns about being too dependent on techniques. What are your concerns on this issue?
4. We take the position that there are more important factors in group work than techniques. If you agree, what do you think these factors are?
5. What do you think about approaching a group with a strict agenda as opposed to letting the group take its own course? Give an example of a population for which an agenda might be appropriate.
6. What are your ideas about using planned group exercises and techniques as a means of stimulating interaction in a group?
7. Give some examples of how and when techniques might interfere with the group process.
8. What are some ways in which you can adapt your techniques to fit the needs of the culturally diverse clients who are likely to be in your groups? How can you create techniques that will accommodate the differences among clients, rather than forcing these clients to fit a predetermined technique? Think of some examples of being inflexible in using techniques with culturally diverse populations.
9. How would you announce to a group that a technique you had introduced was not working?
10. As a group leader, to what degree do you see yourself as structuring and directing the groups you lead, and how would your employment of techniques reflect this structure?
11. We spoke of the importance of the relationship between leader and client. What are some of the ways in which this relationship can be obscured through the use of techniques?
12. How do you view client defenses? Do you see it as appropriate to always break down these defenses?
13. What is your theory of group work, and what is the proper role of techniques in light of that theory?
14. When and how could you explain to a client your rationale for suggesting a technique? What would you not tell a member about a technique?
15. What is your understanding of resistance? Do you see resistance simply as something to be gotten around? Why or why not? Do you see resistance as unwillingness to work? How might you work with resistance?

16. What sorts of techniques would you not use with a psychotic population? an adolescent population? a group of children? a group of elderly persons?
17. We stressed the importance of the personal characteristics of the group leader. What are your thoughts on this matter? What do you see as the most important characteristics for group leaders?
18. Given your own characteristics and experience, why do you think you have a right to counsel others? Suppose a member of a group you were leading asked you this question. What might you say?
19. If you have no faith in group process as a therapeutic agent, how might this attitude affect the outcome for a group you are leading? How might your members sense your attitudes on important matters?
20. Have you participated in a group as a member? What did this experience teach you about yourself? about the group process? about leading groups?
21. What are some ways in which you can best learn which techniques are appropriate and which best fit your personality?
22. What clues do you think would typically form the basis for a hunch of yours about introducing a technique with a particular person?
23. How important is it for you that a technique you introduce work out to be right or appropriate? What inhibits you from trying various techniques?
24. Refer to the ASGW ethical guidelines given in the Appendix, and read them before you go on to Chapter 2. What impressions do you have about these specific guidelines?
25. What topics would you like to have seen added to this chapter, and what would you have said about them?

We suggest that you begin each chapter by reviewing and thinking about the questions at the end. After finishing each chapter, reread the questions, and select the ones you'd like to consider further or discuss in class.

CHAPTER TWO

Ethical Issues in Using Group Techniques

Group Preparation and Norms

The Leader's Motivations and Theoretical Stance

Using Techniques as Avoidance Devices

Undue Pressure

Use of Physical Techniques

Competence in Using Group Techniques

Concluding Comments

Questions and Activities

Before turning to specific techniques, we would like in this chapter to discuss some ethical concerns about using techniques in group work, with a focus on their responsible use. The abuse of techniques does not always stem from a lack of concern for members, for it can arise from a lack of awareness of the potential effects of procedures. We do not attempt to address the broad ethical problems of group work in this chapter. Instead, we are concerned here mainly with specific ethical issues posed by the use of techniques:

- group preparation and norms (providing members with information about the leader, the group's structure and function, and basic policies)
- the leader's motivations and theoretical stance (the possible misuse of techniques for personal reasons and the leader's rationale for the techniques employed)
- using techniques as avoidance devices (such as not dealing with members directly or omitting material with which the leader feels uncomfortable)
- undue pressure (pressure from peers and leaders to participate, misuse of aggressive and confrontational techniques, forced touching, and inappropriate catharsis)
- protecting members when physical techniques are used
- competence in using techniques

In this book we encourage you as a group leader to show spontaneity and inventiveness in the use of techniques. Although we hope that you will develop a level of competence and will trust yourself to devise techniques, you need to strike a balance between this creativity and a healthy caution in using your techniques. From our perspective, the reputation of group counseling has suffered from irresponsible practitioners, mostly those who employ techniques in an ill-conceived or inappropriate way. Our position is that if you have a sound academic background, have had extensive supervised group experience, have acquired some skills in group work, have had your own therapy, and have a fundamental respect for your clients, you are not likely to abuse techniques. However, specific knowledge about the group process and specific skills in facilitating groups are essential for effective group leadership.

Group Preparation and Norms

As we mentioned in the Preface, you will notice that we make frequent reference in this chapter to the ASGW's *Ethical Guidelines for Group Counselors,* because the association has taken the lead in developing a set of professional and ethical guidelines for group practitioners.

Providing information about the group. The ASGW guidelines specify that candidates for group membership have a right to information about the group before they make a commitment to join. Refer to these guidelines in the Appendix for examples of some of the information that potential members should have as a basis for making an informed decision about whether to become a participant.

The techniques appropriate for a group depend on its goals and on the qualifications of the leader. Prospective members and referring agencies should be fully informed about these goals and qualifications. Group leaders should have had academic training in a discipline related to human behavior, in-depth personal therapy or a self-exploration experience, and extensive supervised group work. In addition, it is important that they have a realistic perspective on the limitations of their own training gained from evaluations of their abilities by supervisors and professionals.

In setting group goals and identifying proposed techniques, leaders should be aware that the material they wish to explore should connect with issues that they have looked at in their own lives. And while they may not have experienced every specific technique they intend to use, they should have personally experienced the general procedures they want to employ or should have learned about them under the supervision of someone familiar with them.

As far as is feasible, the kinds of techniques that leaders are likely to employ should be explained to prospective members, and these techniques should be congruent with the leaders' level of training and experience. Leaders should not suppose that the mere possession of relevant academic degrees and licenses guarantees that they are qualified for employing any technique, and they should not suppose that citing such degrees is sufficient to fully inform prospective clients about their qualifications. If the group will emphasize specialized techniques, such as body work, leaders should indicate their qualifications for using these approaches. Leaders who cannot substantiate their training may be misleading prospective clients.

It would be unrealistic to try to explain every technique in advance. But group members can be informed about the general style of the leader. Certainly, if the leader intends to employ highly cathartic techniques such as emotional-release procedures or physical techniques designed to break down resistances, the client should be fully aware of these intentions.

Some of these considerations can be addressed in literature or advertising about the group. One of the best times to inform prospective members about the goals of the group and the training of the leader is during screening and interviewing, which we discuss in the next chapter.

Using tape recordings and videotapes. Recording devices are commonly used as techniques for training purposes and for giving feedback to members. We know of several professors who have not exercised adequate caution in using these training techniques, such as by failing to emphasize confidentiality and to inform students who would have access to these recordings of how they would be used. It is essential that no recordings be made without the knowledge and express consent of the members of the group. Members should know why the session is being recorded or videotaped, what will become of the material, and how it will be used. If the tapes will be used for research or will be listened to or seen and critiqued by a supervisor and students in a practicum, the members have a right to be informed of this use.

Leaders often find it useful to videotape a group session and allow members to view the tape before the next session. Such a tape can eventually be erased, and it can be agreed that it will be used only by the group members and the leaders. If recording devices are used in this way, it is a good policy to inform members that they can stop the machine whenever they feel it is inhibiting their participation.

Perhaps we should note that some members find it difficult to cope with feelings aroused by reviewing alone a recording made of their work in a session. Leaders may want to exercise caution about making such recordings available to members between sessions. In any case, the leader's policies about such matters should be known ahead of time by the prospective members.

The Leader's Motivations and Theoretical Stance

Being aware of motivations.   We are concerned about leaders who use techniques to protect themselves, to meet their own needs for power or prestige, or to control the members of their groups. Group leaders who are unaware of their motivations can misuse techniques in various ways: They may apply pressure on certain clients to get them to perform in desired ways. They may use techniques mainly to impress participants with their therapeutic prowess. They may steer a member away from exploring feelings and issues they personally find threatening. They may use highly confrontive techniques and exercises to stir up aggression in their groups. In all such cases, the leader's needs become primary, while those of the members assume relative unimportance. Although it is certainly acceptable for leaders to have needs, and even to partially meet them through their work in facilitating a group, it is not acceptable for them to exploit members in order to meet these needs.

The potential exists for leaders to hide behind their position. They can camouflage their incompetence, fearfulness, or insecurity by seeking to create the impression that they are all-knowing and all-powerful. They can keep their real feelings hidden and project only what is consistent with the impression they wish to create, and they can choose techniques that perpetuate this illusion.

Even experienced leaders are sometimes slow to recognize such motivations in their use of various techniques. When these abuses become patterns, one can hope that they will show up in the leaders' own therapy or supervised sessions. Co-leaders can also point out these patterns. If leaders do not have supervisors or co-leaders, they should make a habit of reviewing group sessions and staying alert to ways in which their own needs and motives may be getting in the way.

Dealing with the superhuman image.   Group members often attribute exaggerated power and wisdom to leaders, and there is a temptation for leaders who are motivated by a need for power to unethically reinforce this misconception. One way to avoid such reinforcement is to be willing to explain the purpose of a suggested technique. Although it is distracting to explain regularly the point of a technique in advance, at times it might be appropriate for a member to ask about the general purpose of a technique. For instance, Ferdinand said he felt cut off and lonely in the group. When the leader requested that he go into the next room, Ferdinand asked for a reason. Instead of insisting that he "just do it," the leader supplied a brief explanation: "I'd like you to have some sense of what it would be like to accentuate your feeling of being cut off so that we can explore that." At this point the leader might not want to explain certain other reasons for using the technique. For instance, she might have a hunch that Ferdinand was typically sent out of the room as a child and that this exercise would bring back those feelings and allow connections between them and his current loneliness to emerge. The hunch would be sabotaged by explaining it at the beginning, but it might be explained afterward. Explaining techniques in this way tends to discredit the impression that leaders are superhuman wizards. In general, as the trust among the members increases, techniques can be used that are increasingly challenging.

Having a theoretical rationale.   Although leaders can't always predict the exact outcomes of techniques, they can have some idea of how a technique is connected with the material of the moment. If a supervisor, a colleague, or a group member asks a leader "Why did you use that technique? What did you hope to gain from it?" the leader should be able to justify having used it. We are not encouraging leaders to be so preoccupied with thinking about the rationale for a technique that they become timid, but being aware of the purpose of a technique can become second nature and does not have to be incompatible with the ability to follow a hunch spontaneously.

The rationale for using a technique should be rooted in the whole picture of what the client has revealed. Every effort should be made to remember key themes from different episodes in the client's work. For example, one week Bill talked about his fear of becoming involved in an intimate relationship. In another session he was uninvolved in the group; he sprawled in his chair and seemed about to fall asleep. During another meeting, he said he felt he was being treated coldly by others in the group. Remembering these episodes, the group leader attempted to bring them together by inviting Bill to sprawl out and look sleepily around the room, saying to each member a whole sentence that started "A way I keep myself removed from you is . . . " In this example the leader had a rationale: he sought to connect already existing material with the direction the technique was likely to take.

Using Techniques as Avoidance Devices

Avoiding a member's confrontation. In a workshop we witnessed a client attempting to express a legitimate concern to the therapist. The client was asked to pretend that the therapist was in an empty chair and to direct his concerns to the chair rather than to the therapist directly. Such avoidance of dealing directly with a client raises an ethical issue about the therapist's willingness to have honest interaction with clients. It implies that clients have no legitimate issues with the group leader, that what they have to say is only neurotic transference. People cannot enhance their humanness if they are led to believe that their group leaders are better than human.

In another interchange a client expressed anger toward the leader, and the leader responded "I'm glad you can get your feelings out." Such a response is condescending and suggests that the leader is preserving self-esteem at the expense of encountering clients. In supervising student leaders, we sometimes find that they are intimidated by members' anger, especially when it is directed toward them, and that they take steps to bypass angry confrontations. At times their interventions are geared to patching up conflict quickly or avoiding it altogether. For instance, after one angry exchange between two members, one student leader, Herbert, suggested that the two embrace and try to feel "positive feelings" instead of putting each other down. In essence, he asked them to pretend that the conflict did not exist rather than to explore what it was about. As a result of Herbert's discomfort, they did not get to the real issues between them. During the processing time, we focused on Herbert's dynamics that involved his discomfort with any display of anger or conflict. He readily admitted that in his family he had never been allowed to even feel anger, let alone express it openly. He was not clearly aware that the strategies he had introduced during the session were aimed at detouring the members' attempt to work through their conflict. As he talked about what he was feeling and thinking when he was leading, he was able to recognize how his personal limitations were influencing his ability to assist members in dealing with one another honestly.

As the above example shows, when conflict exists within a group, it should be acknowledged directly and dealt with openly. The leader's techniques should not steer members away from what they are feeling but should facilitate direct interaction. If conflict is not brought into the open, it lies dormant and festers, and eventually productive work in the group halts. Unrecognized conflict becomes a hidden agenda, which will certainly interfere with effective group interaction. All too often in everyday life, people are conditioned to skirt the issue of facing and working through conflict. When conflict begins to brew in a group, the natural tendency is to quickly move it aside or to flee from it. Yet this course of action is too familiar, and it really does not teach participants how to successfully work through differences. Members can be challenged to try different behavior in a group setting by making a commitment to continue talking about their reactions to a conflict, rather than to avoid the situation.

Avoiding the leader's fears.   Some leaders introduce techniques to cover up their own fear of exploring the themes that are present in the group. Such diversion frequently occurs when there is distance or hostility in the group.

One of us was supervising a training group in which a student trainee, Pauline, was apparently upset over some unresolved conflict within the group. All of a sudden, she introduced a guided fantasy. Pauline asked members to close their eyes and take a few deep breaths and "just relax." She then guided them to recall a pleasant experience and to see themselves in a place where they very much liked to be. After about ten minutes, one of the members, Sarah, finally exclaimed that she had to talk because she felt as if "I'm going out of my skin." As it turned out, Sarah was angry at Pauline, but she didn't feel that Pauline would allow her to deal with the source of her anger. Soon afterward, almost all of the members began talking about the hostility they had been feeling before Pauline's introduction of the guided fantasy that was aimed at relaxing them. As a result of processing what occurred during this session, the members finally began to open up and express reactions that they had been keeping hidden. Everyone in the group learned how techniques can be used to sabotage a group's effort to develop genuine cohesion by talking out their differences.

If closeness in a group is to be genuine, it takes time to develop. During some periods in a group's history, closeness is often conspicuously absent. If leaders feel afraid, they may try to force a false sense of closeness through the use of various techniques. In one group, for example, the leader suggested that the members huddle together. If any technique was to be introduced, it would have been preferable to suggest that the members of the group spread apart, to far corners of the room, and then be asked to talk about how they felt. In other words, leaders should attempt to make explicit and even exaggerate what is already going on rather than trying to overcome their own fears by imposing an artificial solution.

A related abuse of techniques to avoid the leader's fear often occurs during awkward moments in groups. For example, the group may be lethargic, silences may be long, members may initiate little, and resistance may be manifested in several forms. At times like these we urge leaders to deal directly with this phenomenon. In a desperate attempt to get things moving, some leaders suggest an interaction technique or call on members directly and ask them questions. We think that these techniques cover up potentially rich material. Resorting to techniques to avoid this material is typically a manifestation of leader anxiety.

A broad way of stating the ethical concern here is this: One of the most important things a group teaches is that we can learn to face and express what we think and feel. If group leaders introduce techniques that detract from or cover up the dynamics of the group, they are modeling the idea that our feelings are something to be avoided.

In summary, one should be cautious about using techniques at all if they become substitutes for genuine exploration. In addition, when a technique is introduced, it should generally serve to highlight the cognitive, emotional, and behavioral material present in the group and not to detract from it because of the leader's unease.

Undue Pressure

Freedom not to participate.   Some group leaders make frequent use of interaction exercises, communication exercises, and nonverbal exercises to promote group interaction. For example, a leader may ask members to pair up and engage in a touching exercise or to otherwise express what they are feeling to their partners in a nonverbal way. If leaders are not careful, they can give the impression that all members are expected to participate in all these exercises. Such leaders court the dangers of intruding on clients' sensitivities and of not respecting their right to skip some of the exercises. Some members may feel pressured to do what everyone else is doing, but leaders must make it genuinely acceptable for them to pass by mentioning this option periodically whenever it is appropriate.

To avoid this problem, we usually invite members to work on personally meaningful material. If clients bring up issues they want to explore, the chances are increased that they can handle whatever might surface. Further, we typically impress on members that they can decide at what point they wish to stop. Clients sometimes open up a painful or threatening area and then say that they do not want to go ahead. Generally, we explore their desire for stopping, and in this way we can focus on the factors they find threatening. They may not trust the leader to deal with what will come out. They may not trust the group enough to pursue an issue. They may be worried about looking foolish. Or they may fear losing control and not being able to regain composure. If members do decide to stop, we tell them that if they want to return to the issue later, they should announce this desire. The responsibility is then clearly on the members to decide what they will bring out in the group and the depth to which they will explore the issues they do bring out. Placing responsibility on the members is a built-in safety factor, and it is a sign of our respect for them.

There is another side to this issue. We assume that people who come to a group require some pressure to work effectively. So the task is to achieve a balance between appropriate pressure and unethical coercion. A leader who is reluctant even to say "Are you really sure you are unwilling to do this?" or "How would it be if you just tried this for a minute, and then we could stop if you like?" may be failing to take some responsibility for maintaining a productive environment. Leaders need to be alert to whether a client is leaving an opening for pursuing the technique, but they also have an ethical obligation to respect the client's refusal. Our practice is to respect this refusal and yet to attempt to explore the client's reasons for declining.

In these cases, much depends on the makeup and purpose of a given group, and even more depends on the relationship you have with a particular client. A developed relationship puts you in a position to know where some prodding might be in order. The ethical issue centers on having a basic respect for working with material that is already present and, even more important, a basic respect for the client's decisions about what to explore and how far to go with it.

Pressure from other members.   Group leaders have an ethical obligation to respond to undue peer pressure on a group member, especially when they have assured the group that no one will be coerced into making disclosures or participating in activities. A relevant ASGW guideline on this matter is "Group counselors protect member rights against physical threats, intimidation, coercion, and undue peer pressure insofar as is reasonably possible." A related guideline clarifies the purpose of a group as helping members find their own answers as opposed to pressuring them into doing what the group decides is appropriate. The leader can comment on the peer pressure or can offer an interpretation of the seeming need to coerce and thus can turn the spotlight on the people exerting the pressure. The leader can ask them to talk about why they need to pressure someone else: "You seem intent on getting Jane to talk more. Would you tell her what makes this so important to you?" "Would you tell the group how you are going to feel if you fail to get Jane to do as you wish?" "Would it be relevant for you to talk about relationships you have had outside this group in which you wish someone would do what you are trying to get Jane to do?" The point of such interventions is to acknowledge the feelings of those who are exerting the pressure and to see what productive work might be done with those feelings, while reminding the group of the need to respect the wishes of an unwilling member.

Misuse of confrontational techniques.   At times group leaders can abuse their power by directing techniques toward a particular member. Some leaders derive a sense of power from putting members on the spot and bombarding them with questions or from deliberately putting them in a defensive position. In a group we were supervising, a trainee opened a session by calling on a particular member, and he stayed with this person for the entire session. He believed this was an effective technique to use with resistant clients; he assumed that such pressure would crack their stubborn defenses. Although we think confrontational techniques can be used to work through members' resistances or defenses, we don't think it appropriate to interrogate clients endlessly. When leaders resort to a barrage of questions, the members are likely to close themselves off. Other members tend to pick up the questioning behavior, the atmosphere of trust is lost, and clients are deprived of the opportunity to explore issues in depth. Instead, they think only about how to give appropriate answers to the questions thrown at them. Confrontation needs to be handled with care and concern for the member being confronted.

Forced touching.   There are several facets to the ethical issue of using touching as a technique. In some cases leaders use touching techniques to fulfill their own needs or fantasies and are not sensitive to the needs of group participants. Leaders may have experienced a lack of physical contact in their own lives and may compensate for this lack through their work with groups.

Another ethical aspect of using touching techniques has to do with their potential artificiality. Such techniques can often be used as a shortcut to intimacy. But some clients are not comfortable with being touched or regard a certain level of intimacy as a condition for touching. Because of their cultural background, some clients feel offended at being touched by people with whom they are not intimately acquainted. Some cultures have strong prohibitions against touching between people of opposite sexes. Although increasing some clients' comfortableness with physical contact is therapeutically important, this need should be balanced by respect for the readiness of the participants. We do not discourage spontaneous touching in our groups, but we rarely introduce a technique that explicitly directs clients into a physical intimacy that they do not want. As a group develops intimacy and takes risks, touching tends to increase, but then the touching has been earned rather than imposed. If two members are struggling to get to know each other and to break through their usual boundaries, a touching technique is only likely to bypass the hard work that meaningful intimacy requires.

A final ethical facet of touching arises when a leader is asked to touch someone from whom he or she feels distant. Such a request may arise, for example, when the leader is role-playing a mother or father. Group leaders have an obligation to be genuine in such cases, partly because of the harm that dishonesty has already done to many of their clients. Here the ethical issue is that of being honest with clients and of modeling honesty. Clients are likely to sense when leaders are ignoring their own reservations, and when they do not get straight feedback from the leader, they are deprived of an explanation for the lack of closeness in their lives.

Inappropriate catharsis.   Some leaders are too ready to base the success of their groups on the degree of emotional intensity they evoke and are too eager to push people into a cathartic experience for its own sake. Highly emotional sessions are exciting for their drama, and the expression of emotion is certainly an important component of the group process. The danger is in losing sight of what one hopes to have emerge from catharsis. Moreover, group leaders and members can acquire the expectation that all members should display intense emotion and are somehow failures if they do not do so. We recall a group member who approached a leader during a break and said tearfully that she must not be getting anything from the group because she hadn't yet had a catharsis.

Among the ethical issues that catharsis involves are questions such as these: Whose needs are being met with the catharsis—those of the leader, the group, or the individual member? Is the leader clear about what the catharsis is supposed to mean or lead to? Is the leader capable of handling the intensity of the catharsis or what it might result in? Is there enough time in the group session to work with the emotions that arise and to arrive at a resolution? Will the group leader have subsequent sessions with the client to deal with the repercussions of the catharsis? Is the leader sensitive to the subtle line between invoking catharsis for its therapeutic potential and invoking it for the sake of drama?

Leaders should be especially aware of times when they use catharsis to fulfill their own needs and not those of their clients. The ASGW cautions leaders that their personal and professional needs are not to be met at the members' expense. For example, some leaders may want to see people express anger because they would like to be able to do so themselves, and so they unethically push members to get into contact with angry feelings by developing techniques to bring out such feelings and to focus the group on anger. Certain group therapists can also develop techniques that push members to express only positive and warm feelings toward one another. The point is not that these are illegitimate feelings, for surely most members are at times angry or feeling close. The issue is the degree to which the leader's needs become central in the selection of techniques. This question ought to be raised frequently: "Whose needs are primary, and whose needs are being met—the members' or the leader's?"

Granting the freedom to leave.   Some leaders contend that members should always have the right to leave a group, and others feel strongly that once members have committed themselves to a group, they have an obligation to stay with it. The leader's attitudes and policies about this topic should be spelled out at a preliminary session. On this issue, leaders can be guided by two of the ASGW principles:

> Members have the right to exit a group, but it is important that they be made aware of the importance of informing the counselor and the group members prior to deciding to leave. The counselor discusses the possible risks of leaving the group prematurely with a member who is considering this option.
>
> Before leaving a group, the group counselor encourages members (if appropriate) to discuss their reasons for wanting to discontinue membership in the group. Counselors intervene if other members use undue pressure to force a member to remain in the group.

Our position is that clients have a responsibility to the leaders and the other members of the group to explain why they want to leave. We have several reasons for this policy. It can be deleterious to members to leave without being able to discuss what they considered threatening or negative in the experience. In addition, it is unfortunate for members to leave a group because of a misunderstanding about some feedback they have received. On the other side, it can be damaging to other members if they suppose that someone left the group because of something they said or did. By having the person who is leaving present reasons to the group as a whole, we give the other members an opportunity to verify any concerns they may have about their responsibility for that person's decision. We tell our members that they have an obligation to attend all sessions and to inform us and the group if they intend to miss a session or if they decide to withdraw. If members even consider withdrawing, we encourage them to say so, because such an acknowledgment inevitably provides extremely important material to explore in a session. Although we do not seek to subject members to a debate or to undue pressure to stay, we do stress the serious impact that their leaving will have on the whole group, especially if they do so without explanation. There may be times when a member wants to leave a group, even though the leader is convinced that doing so would not be beneficial for the client. In cases such as this, it is a good practice to offer the person a referral to another source of help.

Use of Physical Techniques

Physical techniques, such as hitting pillows or arm wrestling, often have unpredictable outcomes. The symbolic release of aggression can obviously be valuable, but certain precautions should be taken. Leaders who introduce such techniques should protect the client and the other members from harm and should be prepared to deal with unforeseen directions that the exercise may take. The concern here is not simply for the physical safety of the clients. If a client has restrained emotion for a long time out of fear of the consequences of expressing it, that fear receives tragic reinforcement if the emotion does indeed get out of control when it is expressed and proves damaging to others. In general, we avoid physical techniques involving the whole group for reasons of safety. We prefer to introduce physical techniques only when pursuing work with an individual client with whom we are familiar.

Group counselors who introduce such techniques should have enough experience and training to understand the process and possible consequences of such work. While we encourage leaders to try techniques, we also see a danger in their foolishly or unthinkingly using techniques that they have not experienced themselves or that easily generate material they have no idea how to handle. Merely reading about techniques and then trying them out is not sufficient. Beginning leaders should use them only when direct supervision is available or when they are co-leading with an experienced counselor.

In addition, as we stressed in the previous section, leaders should never goad or push members into physical techniques. Here, inviting members to participate in an exercise and giving them the clear option of refraining are essential. If leaders explain to members the exercise they have in mind, ask them whether they want to try it, and take safety precautions, the chances for negative outcomes are minimized. If physical techniques are occasionally used, it is essential to weigh the potential value of a technique against the potential risk.

Many leaders are interested in a variety of body-oriented techniques that are designed to release intense emotions. These methods typically couple deep or rapid breathing with various postures or movements and combine sounds (moaning or shouting) with the breathing. These techniques are truly powerful, and the intensity they generate can be frightening for the member, or even for the therapist working with such methods for the first time. Additionally, they do have some inherent physical dangers such as hyperventilation.

The central ethical issue is the competence of the leader, an issue we will address further in the next section. The leader who is not ready to deal with strong expressions of emotion ought not to be employing techniques likely to elicit them. A further concern is that the leader be sufficiently familiar with the client to have some basis for judging whether a technique that induces such catharsis is appropriate. These techniques should also be introduced when there is ample time, including follow-up time, for working through the material elicited. We prefer not to employ these techniques to introduce nonexistent feelings, but only to work further with feelings that an individual client is already displaying and ready to intensify. Finally, we try to remember that growth can take place in thoughtful and reflective moments as well as in more overtly emotional situations, so we guard against using physical techniques out of a misplaced need for drama.

Competence in Using Group Techniques

Perhaps the most basic ethical issue pertaining to the use of group techniques is the level of competence achieved by the group worker. Group leaders should not use techniques for which they have not been trained or for which they are not under supervision by a counselor familiar with the intervention. Some other ASGW ethical guidelines regarding the use of techniques are:

- Group counselors should be able to articulate a theoretical orientation that guides their practice and to provide a rationale for their interventions.
- Group counselors should have training commensurate with the potential impact of a technique.
- Group counselors are aware of the necessity to modify their techniques to fit the unique needs of various cultural and ethnic groups.
- Group counselors assist members in transferring learning in the group to daily life.

This issue is not as simple as determining whether someone is a competent group leader or an incompetent one. One needs to consider what competencies are required with what population and with what specific type of group.

One way for you to keep up to date with your knowledge of techniques is to read the professional journals and selected books in group counseling. It is also crucial to do specialized reading about the various populations with which you are working. Simply completing a single course in group counseling as a part of a degree program will not ensure your competence in working with certain challenging populations. Training workshops can upgrade your group-leadership skills.

Students who are in training with us frequently worry whether they know enough to effectively utilize a wide variety of techniques. Although we do not recommend the reckless use of techniques that could open up intensive work for members, we do encourage these trainees to experiment in a safe setting with techniques that are unlikely to lead to work too intense for them to handle. The first principle that we try to get across is the necessity for trainees to experience a wide range of techniques as a member of a group. Merely reading about a technique in a book, observing techniques being used by professionals, or simply discussing techniques does not equip trainees with the skills or the confidence to appropriately and effectively employ techniques. Because we are convinced of the value of certain kinds of experiential group work, we encourage our students to seek out groups in which they can participate fully as a member. This experience has proven invaluable, along with taking courses and getting supervision in training workshops.

Concluding Comments

The most important ethical point we have made in this chapter is that techniques can be harmful if used inappropriately or insensitively. They can injure group participants physically or emotionally. Ethical concerns arise when techniques are used simply as gimmicks and are not designed to serve the needs of the participants. The negative popular image of groups has come from the abuse of techniques, overshadowing the fundamental nature of a group as an arena for genuine and caring human interaction.

Questions and Activities

1. What information should you give potential clients before they enter a group, and what, if anything, should you not inform them about?
2. In order to ethically lead or co-lead a group, what training experiences are necessary? Should being a member in a group be a prerequisite for those who want to lead groups? What kind of group experience would you like to have as a member?
3. Imagine a setting in which a group member declines to participate in a technique or exercise you suggest. Describe how you would respond. How might this refusal have different implications depending on the stage of the group's development?
4. Describe a specific context and client, and explain how you would respond to the client's asking "What is the technique supposed to accomplish?"
5. We hold that leaders should have a theoretical rationale to support their choice of a technique. Do you agree? Think of some specific techniques

you have used in leading a group. What was your rationale for using them?

6. Think of a situation in which a conflict is not being openly expressed within a group. What do you think you would do? How might using a technique in this situation mask your fears about your competence?

7. How do you teach your group members to confront in a constructive manner? What are the differences between confrontation and attack?

8. Do you think that psychological risks are necessarily a part of group participation? Explain. What are some specific risks related to participating in a group? Can you think of safeguards that are likely to minimize risks?

9. A client is following a technique that you have introduced and then says that she wants to stop. Would you be inclined to explore with her the reasons for wanting to stop? Why or why not?

10. Under what circumstances and conditions do you believe it appropriate for a member to leave a group? Explain your position.

11. How would you explain to a group the importance of confidentiality? Are there any techniques you might use in connection with this explanation?

12. What are some ways in which techniques might be misused that we have not talked about?

13. Describe what you regard as unethical motivations for using a technique.

14. As a leader, what advantages do you see to being self-disclosing? What are some ways in which a group leader might hide behind his or her professional role?

15. A member says to you: ''I don't know you. I want to have you share more of yourself personally so that I can trust you.'' How might you respond?

16. What are your thoughts about the kind of continuing education that you would like as a way to upgrade your skills in group leading?

17. What considerations do you think are important in deciding whether a leader should touch a client?

18. Explain your position on planned exercises involving touching. How would you deal with a situation in which one or more members objected to being touched? If you did introduce exercises involving touching, what would be your reasons for doing so?

19. You find yourself introducing many techniques involving physical touching and physical closeness. How would you try to determine whether you were mainly meeting your own needs or responding to material that the group wanted to explore?

20. What are some considerations involved in adapting techniques to the needs of culturally diverse populations? How might you modify certain techniques to fit the needs of clients who are culturally different from you?

21. You observe that several members of your group are pressuring an individual to say or do something. How do you think you might respond in this situation?
22. Do you think you should have experienced a technique yourself before you introduce it in a group? Explain.
23. We have urged you to be cautious on a number of grounds, and we have also encouraged you to be creative in your use of techniques. What would you describe as your own guidelines for reconciling these two seemingly contradictory suggestions? When should creativity yield to caution?
24. In what ways can you ethically fulfill your own desires and needs while you are a leader of a group? What problems do you see if you rely on your work as a group leader to meet your needs?
25. Explain what you believe to be the most important ethical considerations regarding group techniques. Are there any that we have failed to discuss in this chapter?

CHAPTER THREE

Techniques for Preparing Groups

$\mathbf{I}$n this chapter we share some of the ways we have found for getting groups established. We describe techniques for recruiting, screening, selecting, and preparing members for effective work. Clients have a right to know the goals and procedures of a group, and they should be informed about their rights and responsibilities as members and the expectations that leaders have for them. Participants will get the most from their group experience if leaders do some teaching about the group process at the beginning. We find that if members are inadequately prepared, the group typically gets stuck in the initial stage because the participants are unable to work through conflicts that result from a lack of basic information. In our view, using the techniques described in this chapter is one of the best ways of ensuring that a group will move forward.

Getting Groups Established

A demanding part of conducting groups is the work you do before the first session. In an organized setting—a school, a mental-health agency, a mental hospital, a clinic—you will usually need approval to organize a group. In such situations you will find it helpful to write a proposal that clarifies your goals. If the goals are vague, neither your administrator nor the potential members will be likely to receive the idea for a group enthusiastically. With a well-thought-out proposal you can sell potential participants or directors on the value of a group program. In addition, a carefully written proposal can prevent the confusion and misunderstanding that often derail groups.

In writing a proposal, you should consider the following questions:

- What are your qualifications for leading the group, and how can you best present your background experience?
- What kind of group will this be? What structure will the group have?
- What will be your major functions as group leader?
- Why is a group useful for the purposes you hope to accomplish? What are the unique properties of a group that make it valuable for your particular population?
- For whom is the group designed?
- What will be the main goals of the group?
- Where will the group be held? How long will it last?
- What topics do you expect to be explored?
- How will you deal with the potential dangers or risks of group participation?
- What evaluation procedures will you use to determine the degree to which the group has met its goals? What assessment procedures can you devise to help members monitor the degree to which they are satisfied with their participation in the group?
- What follow-up procedures will you use to help members integrate what they have learned and evaluate this learning?

• • • • • • • • • • • • • • • • • • • •

Designing a Time-Limited Group: An Illustration*

I regularly offer a 16-week group in my private practice. What follows is a description of the purpose and framework of this group, along with suggestions for orienting members and shaping specific group norms.

Rationale for the time limitation. This group provides an example of strategies for teaching clients to become active in deciding what they want to change in their life and strategies for providing them with the tools to practice alternative behaviors. Limiting the time frame of the group frequently stimulates members to determine whether they are fully investing themselves. It is not assumed that the length of therapy is equated with its effectiveness. Some popular forms of cognitive-behavioral therapy design 10- to 16-week treatment programs geared to produce change. Apart from theoretical support for shorter groups, there is another and more pragmatic reason for the reduced time. Practitioners who work with less affluent populations know the difficulty of requiring a commitment of time and money from them. It is beyond the means of many people to commit to attending a group every week for 12 months or longer. For those who are not psychologically sophisticated, a relatively long-term group may seem like a greater commitment than they are willing to make, especially when they are approaching a group experience with hesitation.

   I do not mean to imply that the 16-week group is an inferior form of therapy that is geared toward the less affluent. Sixteen-week groups have many beneficial factors working in their favor. Any practitioner of group therapy has to be aware of the "cozy-nest syndrome" that groups can provide. Some people succumb to it and stay endlessly in group therapy, always "working" and perhaps never changing. The 16-week group confronts members with the necessity of *doing* something in the group and also taking action outside of the group to change their lives. The members need to determine whether they are seriously committed to changing their lives.

Key features in the group's formation. This group is composed of people with a variety of personal and interpersonal problems that have prompted them to seek a therapist. The participants may have difficulty in developing and maintaining close relationships. They may have a range of bodily symptoms. They may have come to the realization that their life is dull, without any seasoning. Although their problems are not severe enough to require medication or hospitalization, the members often feel "stuck" and are seeking a group experience as a way of helping them make some new decisions. Below are some of the key features in designing this group:

• Attendance is stressed. If people come and go at will in a group, there is a reduction of intensity and a low level of trust. It is difficult to trust group

*This section is written from the perspective of Patrick Callanan.

members when they treat their commitment in a casual way. If a member expects to miss 3 or more sessions out of 16, it is usually best to ask the person to withdraw from the group.

- Members are reminded that they are in the group to find out something about themselves, not primarily to get close to people, to make friends, or to avoid loneliness.
- Clients are told that they should actively attempt to behave differently than they typically do. The group provides some degree of safety for them to experiment with change, but in a 16-week group, time is short.
- The group has eight members, it meets for two hours, and the members determine the agenda for the sessions as the group progresses. In addition to the weekly meetings, an extended session of six hours is scheduled at some point. This provides an opportunity to do more intensive work.

A Contrasting Approach: The Long-Term Group*

In contrast to time-limited groups, such as the one just described, I am especially interested in long-term groups. This format is exemplified by a psychoanalytic group I have been co-leading with my wife, Sandra Russell. We hope to create an environment that helps members understand and modify their unconscious contributions to their present conflicts, which have their paradigms in infantile separation and individuation and oedipal rivalry. Many of the techniques for this format arise from our efforts to achieve a stable group environment and then to interpret reactions to events that threaten this stability. Contrary to our usual practice of distributing written information to members at the formation of a group, in this case we have not done so. This is partly because most of the original members of this group were themselves either therapists or persons with considerable sophistication in therapy, and we wanted to see what group norms and expectations would evolve in the absence of explicit written directives. Most of the members had previous experience in shorter intensive groups, and they typically felt they had made considerable headway with specific behavioral objectives but wanted a better grasp of persisting underlying character dynamics. For this group, rather than distribute literature, we held one or more individual screening meetings, explaining that we were seeking to provide a long-term group relationship in which members could draw from an extensive history with one another to get insight into themes developing over time.

We explained to prospective clients that they were being asked to join the group only if they would commit to remaining for at least a year. We told them that when they paid for their first meeting, they were also to put on deposit payment for their eventual last two sessions. This prepayment was required to underscore a commitment to attend for a minimum of two weeks after giving notice of their intention to terminate. We also told them that as long as they were occupying a place in the group, they were expected to pay for each session, even if they could not attend. And we asked them to

*This section is written from the perspective of Michael Russell.

call ahead to notify the group if they were going to be absent. These policies tend to accentuate the awareness that members have about the group as an important entity. The prospect of members' joining or leaving this group is inevitably an occasion for an in-depth examination of feelings such as the stability of the infantile maternal environment, which the group represents, or fears that established means of gaining "parental" attention will be disrupted.

The main point is that there is considerable latitude in how you might set up the ground rules for a group, depending on your objectives, population, and theoretical orientation.

• • • • • • • • • • • • • • • • • • • •

Having described some differences between designing a time-limited group and a long-term group, we now move to a discussion of specific techniques that you may find useful in forming a variety of groups. In the remaining sections we consider strategies for recruiting, screening, selecting, and preparing members for a group. Our focus is on the importance of the preliminary group session for orientation purposes and on techniques for assisting members in defining and clarifying their personal goals. We also list guidelines and suggestions for members to derive the maximum benefit from a group.

Recruiting Members

Personal contact is the best way to recruit potential candidates for a group, because members are committing themselves to working with a specific person. In addition, through personal contact the leader can enthusiastically demonstrate that the group has potential value for a person.

Rather than simply relying on flyers, leaders can contact people who might direct clients to them: colleagues, directors of clinics, teachers and professors, physicians, ministers, school counselors, psychologists, and social workers. It is a group leader's responsibility to become familiar with the resources in the community. This implies a willingness to educate referral sources. Indeed, this is probably the best method of recruiting potential group members.

In the recruitment process, potential clients have a right to know the goals of the group, the basic procedures to be used, what will be expected of them as participants, what they can expect of the leader, and any major risks as well as potential values of participating in the group.

Screening and Selecting Members

The next step is to determine who might profit from the group and who (if anyone) should be excluded. One technique for making these decisions is to meet privately with every person who wishes to join the group. In such a meeting the leader can get a sense of the appropriateness of including particular candidates and can give them a chance to determine whether they want to be involved. Leaders need to keep in mind that all groups are not appropriate for all people. Indeed, for some, group participation can be damaging or at least counterproductive to their growth. The question of the appropriateness of including a member is directly related to the purpose and goals of the group. Let's assume that a candidate for a group, Wilma, meets with the therapist for a half-hour individual screening session. She can also ask questions of the leader to help her determine if she wants to be in this group. Ideally, the interview will be a two-way exchange in which a mutual decision is made. The leader can ask questions such as the following of Wilma to get a sense of her readiness for the group:

- "Why do you want to join the group?"
- "How ready are you to take a critical look at your life?"
- "What would you most hope to get from the group? Will this group help you achieve your goals?"
- "What do you want to know about me?"
- "Do you understand the purposes and nature of the group?"
- "What are some specific personal concerns that you'd most like to explore?"

This individual contact between the prospective member and the leader can be extremely useful as a way to begin to establish trust, for it can allay fears and provide the foundation for future work. Of course, orientation interviews are time consuming and may not always be feasible, but they are worth the time that they take. Even a brief contact significantly reduces risk and contributes to the overall quality of the group. This contact provides members with some idea of what to expect, and thus they are more likely to come prepared to work.

Sometimes it is impossible to individually screen prospective members. For instance, you may work in a residential facility, so that your groups are formed on the basis of people who live on the same ward. When screening is not possible, it is important to devise some alternative strategy. At least you can meet with individuals on the ward before they are placed in your group and orient them to the process. If time constraints make it impractical for you to screen each member individually, you can experiment with group interviews.

Conducting a Preliminary Session

In addition to an individual meeting before selection for membership in the group, we recommend a preliminary session with the potential members. The primary purpose of this meeting is for the leader to outline the aims of the group in detail and to clarify what the participants will be doing. It gives participants an opportunity to meet one another and to get additional data for making their decision about committing themselves to the group.

Such a meeting has the following specific purposes: getting acquainted; clarifying personal goals and group goals; learning about the procedures to be used in the group; learning about how the group will function and how to get the most from the experience; discussing the possible dangers or risks involved in participating in the group and ways of minimizing these risks; discussing the essential requirement of confidentiality and any other necessary ground rules; exploring with members their fears, expectations, hopes, and ambivalent feelings; and answering their questions. During this pregroup meeting, members sometimes have few questions, and in those cases we tend to raise questions that we know are frequently on the minds of people who are about to enter a group. Examples of questions that members have brought to a preliminary session are:

- "Will I be pushed to go further than I feel comfortable?"
- "Is everything that we say in the group to be held confidential?"
- "If I get scared, is it acceptable to leave a session?"
- "Will you, as group leaders, be sharing with us personally, and will you also be group members?"
- "What kind of techniques are likely to be a part of this group?"
- "What are some problems that people typically bring with them to a group such as this?"
- "How will I know if I fit in this group?"

At the end of the first session, clients can be asked to think about whether they still want to join the group. A leader who has reservations about admitting a member can arrange for another interview to explore these reservations.

Let's look at specific matters that need to be openly explored at the preliminary session (and then again perhaps during the initial meeting). One is confidentiality. Members will not feel free to explore issues in a meaningful way if they don't have the assurance that what they say will be held in confidence by both the leaders and the other members. Members need to be reminded emphatically about how easily they may unintentionally breach the confidences of other members by talking about specifics brought up in the group. And leaders must state directly and openly any limitations of confidentiality. They should inform members of the circumstances under which they will have to divulge material that is brought up in the group. Such a statement is especially important in a mandatory group in a detention facility. For example, if a group leader must report on the clients' progress, he or she should clearly point out this requirement and make it a topic for discussion. There are other limitations of confidentiality, such as the legal requirement to report cases of suspected child abuse or incest or to report situations involving potential harm to the client or others.

Other basic matters that might be mentioned at the preliminary session include policies on matters such as smoking or eating in the group, coming to the group on time, missing group sessions, socializing outside the group and other subgrouping matters, and having sessions recorded.

The best technique is for the leader to simply state some essential procedures and policies and discuss them in the group. In addition, the leader can distribute two copies of a list of the important group procedures and policies to each member. Members can sign both copies, keeping one and giving the other to the group leader. Leaders who use this technique as a way of clarifying and focusing on procedures and policies should go over the policies with the members and express the reasons for establishing them. Following is a typical list of ground rules for a group.

• • • • • • • • • • • • • • • • • •

Ground Rules

1. Members are not to use drugs or alcohol during a session and are not to come to a session under the influence of any chemical agents.
2. Members are expected to be present at all the group meetings, because their absence affects the entire group.
3. Members must avoid sexual involvement with others in the group during its duration.
4. Members are not to use physical violence in group sessions, nor are they to be verbally abusive to others in the group.
5. Members will be given a summary of their rights and responsibilities so that they know what is expected of them before they join the group.
6. Members must keep confidential what other members do and say within the group.

• • • • • • • • • • • • • • • • • •

Because of time constraints, a preliminary session may not be feasible in all cases, even though it is highly recommended. As a substitute, group leaders can integrate many of the ideas we cover here into the first session. The initial group meeting can then be an orientation session during which members decide whether the group is appropriate for them. Even if your group meets for as few as six sessions, some type of preliminary orientation session would be very helpful. We suggest adding one session for this preliminary preparation of members.

Preparing Parents of Minors

In planning a group composed of children or adolescents, it is generally wise to contact the parents of the potential members and secure their written permission before allowing the members to enroll in the group. However, the practice of informed consent and of getting parental permission for counseling services varies from school to school and from state to state.

An additional technique is to invite parents and their children to a meeting with you so that you can present the need for such a group and discuss their questions or concerns. Sending letters to parents and holding a meeting with them and their children can prevent many problems from developing later. If parents are not informed or their cooperation is not enlisted, conflicts may result. Your presentation can put to rest some of the false notions that parents may have about the group. For example, some parents may think that family matters will be publicly aired or that their children will be brainwashed.

Setting Goals

Members and leaders should set goals for themselves, both at the start of a group and at the start of each session, if maximum learning is to occur. Members can begin to set these goals at the screening interview and also at the preliminary session. We describe in this section some techniques the leader may want to use in this process. We hope that you will not consider the activities we describe as school assignments but as focusing methods. These are merely suggestions to choose from, and you would not want to use all these techniques in one group.

The kind of preparation we discuss here can be used in any group but is particularly useful in giving direction to groups, such as those for children, that need a significant degree of structure in order to function effectively. A balance needs to be maintained between too much structure and not enough. Too much structure may squelch the creativity and self-direction of group members, and not enough preparation may cause a group to flounder needlessly because of a lack of focus. Another factor to consider in deciding on the degree of structure is the leader's experience, training, and personal characteristics. Some leaders work better with more structure, some with less.

A leader will have goals in mind for a group. These can be general goals that have to do with establishing an environment within which members can attain their personal goals. And they can be process goals such as learning appropriate self-disclosure, being willing to share feelings, being willing to talk in a personal way, staying in the here and now, expressing reactions to what is going on in the group, learning how to confront with care and respect, and learning how to give others feedback. If members know these goals from the start, they have a clear idea of what is expected of them and also how they might get the most from the group for themselves.

In addition, members should clarify what they want from a group. Their thinking on this matter is often fuzzy and global. They hope to get in touch with their feelings, they would like to communicate better, or they want to work on understanding themselves. These vague goals are hard to work on in a group. Helping members translate them into specific ones is the first step in preparation. Thus, if a member says "I want to learn how to express my feelings," the leader might ask: "What particular feeling do you have the most trouble expressing? In what situations do you find it most difficult to express this feeling? What's it like for you to be this way? How would you like to be different?"

Asking members to tell one another of their specific goals is one way to get them to think about their reasons for being in the group. Having them write down these goals is valuable. One technique that some of our student leaders have used in their groups is to ask their members at the first session to write a letter to themselves, which will be opened at the last meeting. The participants are asked to write a paragraph on what they would most like to say that they had gotten out of the group experience. At the final session, the members unseal their letters and decide whether to share with others what they wrote to themselves. A variation is to ask people to write down at an early session what they hope to have done, whom they hope to have become, or how they hope to have changed in six months or a year. They give these statements to the leader in self-addressed, stamped envelopes, and the leader mails them unopened at the end of the time period. Not only do such exercises challenge members to look at what they want for themselves, but they are also a device for accountability. These letter techniques can be useful in helping members get a focus on what they want from a group experience as well as what they would like to do in applying this experience to their everyday lives.

Preparing contracts.   A full contract is an extension of the letter-writing techniques. In contracts members write out the specific behaviors or attitudes they want to change and what they are willing to do inside and outside the group to make these changes. Members can compose these contracts at home after the first session, bring them back to the group at the second meeting, and discuss them in the group. The leader and other members can offer their perceptions of how realistic the person's goals are and can offer other ways to meet the objectives. Following are some guidelines to assist in designing contracts. An effective contract is:

- concise and specific
- stated in behavioral terms
- realistic and attainable
- broken into short-term and long-term goals
- related to the general goals and purpose of the group

Contracts should not be compared to legal documents; rather, they provide a strategy for helping members be specific about those thoughts, feelings, and actions they would like to change. The contract can spell out how they intend to make the change, a schedule for doing so, and possible strategies for coping with setbacks to their plans.

Reading.   Depending on the kind of group, reading can be a great asset to the members. By doing some reading before the group begins, participants solidify their commitment and focus. Reading can assist them in reflecting on their lives and on what they want to change. For example, for an assertiveness-training group, the members can read a popular treatment that discusses typical situations in which people encounter difficulties and ways to act in these situations assertively.

Reading can be used as a focusing technique in other ways. You may be aware of a specific theme that a particular member of the group plans to explore and be able to recommend a book that helps the member focus on that topic. You may also ask members to select from among the many self-help paperbacks ones that they expect might be useful for them. Or you may give them a bibliography about groups or about probable group topics and urge them to select ones that they think might be especially meaningful at this point in their lives. You may also encourage group participants to reread a book that has had an impact on them or to reread their favorite childhood fairy tale and reflect on whether it symbolized any struggles they faced. Reading can prime people to think about issues in their lives that they would like to bring to a group. It is also a way of getting people to continue working between sessions.

Writing journals.   Writing can be used in several ways as an adjunct to preparation for a group or for a specific meeting. Members can spend ten minutes each day recording in a journal certain feelings, situations, behaviors, and ideas for courses of action. For example, clients who are working at being assertive and speaking out can make journal entries about the inner dialogue they have before deciding to express an idea, about times they did express an opinion (how they felt, how others reacted to them), about times they sat quietly thinking they had nothing valuable to offer (and how they felt then), and about how to change these patterns.

Members can also review certain periods of time in their lives and write about them. For example, they can get out pictures of their childhood years and other reminders of this period and then freely write in a journal whatever comes to mind. Writing in a free-flowing style without censoring can be of great help in getting a focus on feelings.

Members can bring the journals to the group and share a particular experience they had that resulted in problems for them. They can then explore with the group how they might have handled the situation better. In general, however, these journals are for the benefit of the members, to help them focus themselves for a session. The members themselves can decide what they do with the material they write.

Another way to use journals is as a preparation for encountering others in everyday life. For instance, Jenny is having a great deal of difficulty talking with her husband. She's angry with him much of the time over many of the things he does and does not do. But she sits on this anger, and she feels sad that they don't take time for each other. Jenny typically doesn't express her sadness to him, nor does she let him know of her resentment toward him for not being involved in their children's lives. To deal with this problem, she can write her husband a detailed and uncensored letter pointing out all the ways in which she feels angry, hurt, sad, and disappointed and expressing how she would like their life to be different. It is not necessary that she show this letter to her husband. The letter writing is a way for her to clarify what she does feel and to prepare herself to work in the group. This work can then help her to be clear about what she wants to say to her husband as well as how she wants to say it. This process works in the following way: Jenny can say aloud some of what she wrote to a member in the group who role-plays her husband. Others can then express how they experience her and the impact she has on them. Aided by such feedback, she may be able to hit on a constructive way of expressing her feelings to her husband in real life.

Still another technique is for members to spontaneously enter in their journals their reactions to themselves in the group:

- How do I feel about being in this group?
- How do I see people in the group? How do I see myself in it?
- How do I sabotage myself so that I don't get what I might from this group? How can I challenge myself when I become aware of defeating myself?
- What are some ways in which I resist? How do I avoid things?

If people write down their reactions in this way, they are likely to verbalize them in the group. For instance, if members fear opening up lest others see them as being stupid, this fear prevents them from sharing their concerns. If they write about this fear and then bring it up for consideration in the group, they lessen their chances of being stopped by the fear.

Another useful technique is for people to write down their reactions to each session. A brief review of the session provides them with a running account of their experiences in the group. As the group is coming to an end, these notes can be useful in recalling and understanding specific events.

Writing can be useful as the group progresses as well as during the early stage. At the midpoint of a group, people can take time during the week to write down how they feel about the group at this point, how they view their participation in it so far, what they are doing outside the group to attain their goals, and how they'd feel if the group were to end now. By discussing these statements in the group, participants are challenged to reevaluate their level of commitment and are often motivated to increase their participation in the group.

In training group leaders, we encourage them to make frequent journal entries about themselves and the reactions that are evoked in them as they are leading or co-leading their groups. Rather than describing the dynamics of their members, we suggest that they focus on how specific members affect them personally. The following questions are some of the ones that we recommend that group leaders address in their journals:

- How did I feel about myself as I was leading or co-leading my group?
- What did I like best about the group today?
- What most stood out for me during this session?
- How am I being affected personally by each of the members?

- How involved am I in this group?
- Are there any factors that are getting in the way of my effectively leading this group?

The use of the journal technique for group leaders provides and excellent record of patterns that are shaping up in a group. The practice of writing can also be a useful catalyst for focusing leaders on areas in their own lives that need continued attention.

Using structured questionnaires. A sentence-completion questionnaire that includes the following statements might be administered to a group in an early session:

- What I most want from this group is . . .
- The one thing I'd most want to be able to say at our final meeting is . . .
- Thinking about being in this group for the next 20 weeks, I . . .
- A fear I have about being a group member is . . .
- One personal concern I would hope to bring up is . . .
- I often feel . . .
- The one aspect I'd most like to change about myself is . . .
- Something I particularly like about myself is . . .

This is a focusing device, and it can be followed with a discussion of whatever it brings out in the members.

A problem checklist is another valuable tool for helping members decide how they want to use the group time. For example, for an adolescent group you can develop a list of problems that teenagers typically face, and members can write down the degree to which each problem applies to them (anonymously if they wish). The following inventory is an illustration.

• • • • • • • • • • • • • • • • • • • •

Problem Checklist for an Adolescent Group

Directions: Rate each of the following problems as they apply to you at this time, and indicate (by using one of the numbers 1, 2, 3, below) the degree to which you'd like help from the group with them:

(1) This is a major problem for me, one I hope will be a topic for exploration in the group.
(2) This is a problem for me at times, and I could profit from an open discussion of the matter in this group.
(3) This is not a concern of mine, and I don't feel a need to explore the topic in the group.

- feeling accepted by my peer group
- learning how to trust others
- getting along with my parents (brothers, sisters)
- getting a clear sense of what I value

- worrying about whether I'm "normal"
- being fearful of relating to the opposite sex
- dealing with sexual feelings, actions, and standards of behavior
- being so concerned about doing what is expected of me that I don't live by my own standards
- worrying about my future
- wondering whether I will get into college
- trying to decide on a career

Additional problems I'd like to pursue:

_____

_____

_____

• • • • • • • • • • • • • • • • • • • •

A questionnaire does not have to be this elaborate. In an adolescent group, for example, one could simply ask: "What problems would your parents like you to discuss in this group, and what would you like to say about these problems? What issues might your peers suggest to you for exploration in this group?"

Constructing a critical-turning-points chart. Another technique to prepare members for productive work is asking them to draw a road map of their lives and include some of the following points of interest: key turning points, major crises, big decisions, new opportunities, major accomplishments, severe failures, important people, and major disappointments. Members can then work in pairs, selecting whatever they would like to share from their charts. Or they can talk about critical turning points in their lives with the entire group. In addition to or in place of a chart, clients can draw a sketch divided into three parts: "My Past/My Present/My Future." Much of their drawing may be symbolic. Again they can share what parts of their sketch mean to them in small groups or in the group as a whole.

Writing an autobiography. Another technique for getting members focused is to ask them to write autobiographies in which they present their current subjective views of various points in their lives: childhood, adolescence, early adulthood. They can be encouraged to stress significant events, persistent emotions, dreams, relationships with others, and parallels in their lives at present. They might pay particular attention to those events that evoked intense emotions, because these may contain clues to work they decide to pursue in the group. It helps to ask members not to write merely factual accounts of their lives but, instead, to focus on the personal meaning that certain events had for them. For example, a male member may write about ways in which his parents' divorce affected him during his adolescence.

He may talk about feeling guilty and responsible for the breakup of his parents. Another member, a young woman, may write about how incest during her adolescence continues to influence her as an adult. Another member may talk about a midlife career change that she made and the flak that she received from her family. She could write about how the negative reactions from her children and husband are still affecting her. The useful feature of writing autobiographies is that core material can be brought into group sessions for further exploration.

Using fantasy. An open-structured or nondirective fantasy technique can be useful in the early stages of a group for individual focusing, for providing data, and for getting group members acquainted with one another. One such exercise, which can be done either in writing or orally, goes like this: "Imagine that you are a book. What's a good title for you that captures something of what you are all about? What's your style, your tone? What are your chapter headings? How about your cover and your preface—will people be enticed to read you? Are you going to deliver what you advertise? Which chapters of you were the hardest to write? Which chapters would you want to have deleted? After people have read through you, cover to cover, what do you suppose they will think?"

The same device can be used during the ending stages of a group when members are being asked to consolidate their group experience: "Thinking back to the book you imagined yourself to be at the beginning of this group, do you want now to have a different title? What other changes and revisions would you like to make, from beginning to end?"

Preparing Members to Get the Most from a Group

At the initial session you can discuss with members some guidelines for involving themselves in the group and applying what they learn to their daily lives. In order to gain the most from a group, participants need to be oriented and prepared. Of course, there is a danger in overpreparing members. By spending too much time teaching them what to look for and how to act, you run the risk of doing too much of the work that the group ultimately needs to do for itself. Even though not every possibility should be covered, some preparation at the outset can create a climate conducive to productive work as the group moves into its advanced stages. In many ways, the norms that govern group behavior are foreign to the expected behavior in daily living. Group members are expected to express feelings, to ask directly for what they want, to take time for themselves, to allow themselves to be vulnerable, to tell others how they affect them, to deal with conflict, and to make decisions for themselves. Many of these behavioral standards are contrary to the process of socialization that most of us have experienced. Members need to acquire a mind set for how to actively participate in an interpersonal group. All this preparation doesn't have to be completed at the initial session. Much of it needs to be reinforced and discussed during the first few meetings.

The best way to distribute this information is to write it down and give it to members at the screening interview, the preliminary session, or the first group session. The following guidelines are designed for growth groups for relatively well-functioning adults. The list can be shortened or modified depending on the specific population and the type of group.

• •

Guidelines and Suggestions for Group Members

1. *Have a focus.* Commit yourself to getting something from this group by focusing on what you hope to accomplish. In clarifying your goals, review specific issues you want to explore, specific changes you want to make, and actions you are willing to take to make these changes. Before each group session, take time to clarify what you would like to bring up during that meeting, and write these issues down if that is helpful to you.

2. *Be flexible.* Although it helps to approach a group session with some idea of what you want to explore, don't be so committed to your agenda that you can't work with what comes up spontaneously within the group. Be open to pursuing alternative paths if you are affected by others in your group.

3. *Don't wait to work.* It is easy to let a group session go by without getting around to what you hope to do or say. The longer you wait to involve yourself, the harder it will become. Therefore, challenge yourself to have something to say at the beginning of each group, even if it's a brief statement of what it was like for you to come to the group that day.

4. *Be ''greedy.''* The success of a group depends on your being eager to do your own work. This doesn't mean that you should monopolize time or be insensitive to the difficulty others may have in getting into the spotlight. But if you constantly wait until it's your "turn" or try to monitor how much of the group's time should be allotted to you, you will inhibit the spontaneity and enthusiasm that can make a group exciting and productive. If each member takes responsibility for pursuing his or her own work, everyone should have enough opportunity to speak.

5. *Pay attention to feelings.* Intellectual discussions are great, but an experiential group is about your feelings and convictions. If you do nothing but expound your theories and opinions, you will not explore your life on an emotional level. As a rule of thumb, if your sentences can just as well start "My opinion is that . . . ," you probably are not working much on a feeling level, and you are not taking full advantage of the unique opportunity for doing so that an experiential group provides. You don't need to work hard to generate feelings, but be open to letting yourself experience them as you are in a session and as you are present for others. Also, if you are talking about a topic in the group, find some way to show how this matter is connected with you personally. Avoid abstract discussions of topics that have no personal relevance.

6. *Express yourself.* Most of us are in the habit of censoring our expression of thoughts and feelings. We are afraid of being inappropriate or, often, afraid that we will simply magnify and entrench the feelings and convictions we have if we voice them. These fears are not unfounded, but we have far more reason to be concerned about what we do to ourselves when we don't verbalize than when we do. And experientially there is a world of difference between thinking something through in our minds and saying it out loud. A group is an ideal place to find out what would happen if we expressed what we felt, which can be a powerful and positive experience. If you have feelings that relate to the group, be willing to express them. For example, if you are aware of feeling bored, announce that you feel this way, and be willing to take responsibility for your own boredom. "Sitting on feelings" is a sure way to dam up the flow of a group.

7. *Be an active participant.* You will help yourself most if you take an active role in the group. Silent observers are not likely to get as much from their participation in the group, and others may believe that their silence means they are being judgmental. Although silent members may be learning vicariously, they deprive others of the opportunity to learn from them. Realize that others will not know you if you remain silent on issues that are important to you. At least let people know what it is like for you to be in a particular group session. Even if you did not do any focused work yourself during the session, you are likely to have had reactions to what went on with others. Let them know how their work affected you.

8. *Experiment.* Look at the group as a place in which you are relatively safer and freer than usual to express yourself in different ways and to try out different sides of yourself. Having done so, you can then seek ways of carrying these new behaviors into your outside life. In between group meetings, think of specific ways in which you can practice and experiment with the behaviors you are acquiring in your group. Then, report to the group how you are letting yourself behave differently outside.

9. *Grow.* Groups are built on the assumption that no matter how well your life may be going now, it can be enriched by the opportunity to explore your feelings, values, beliefs, attitudes, and thoughts and to consider changes you may want to make. If you believe that such exploration is appropriate only for people with severe emotional problems, you are shortchanging yourself and the other participants. Even though you do not have any pressing crisis in your life, assume that the issues that come up for you are worth exploring.

10. *Don't expect change to be instantaneous.* If you do seek to change some features of your life, remember that such changes do not usually happen all at once or without some backsliding. Don't be overly critical of yourself if you experience setbacks. Realize that it will take time to change long-standing patterns and that there may be a tendency to revert to familiar ways when you are faced with stressful situations. Give yourself credit for what you are willing to try and for subtle changes you can see yourself making.

11. *Don't expect others to appreciate your changes.* Some people in your life may have a considerable investment in keeping you the way you are now. Expect to find less support outside the group than within it for your struggles, and use the group as a place to explore some of the resistance you encounter outside. It is a good idea to remind yourself that you are in this group primarily to make the changes that you want in yourself, not to change someone else. It may happen that you come to understand others more fully or that others in your life change in response to your being different, but don't focus on them primarily.

12. *Don't expect to be understood within the group.* Groups heighten a sense of intimacy and provide an opportunity for being understood by others in ways we don't always experience in our daily lives. But in many respects you simply will not be understood by the others in your group. They will see certain dimensions of you but will not have a good idea of what you are like otherwise. If you are working mainly on conflicts or emotional vulnerability, the group will see this side of you. You can waste your time and everyone else's if you feel you must constantly qualify and footnote everything you express. A concern that everyone get the full picture—which probably is impossible anyway—will just distract you from achieving your goals in the group. For example, if you choose to explore some feelings you have about a relationship you are in and think you must explain those feelings by giving a full and "objective" account of the relationship, you will be talking forever. Better to resign yourself in advance to the idea that others won't and can't have the full picture.

13. *Don't expect to understand others in the group.* The other side of this point is that you do a disservice to others in the group if you suppose that you have them all figured out. Like you, they are presumably working on expressing a side of themselves that they do not usually have an opportunity to express. If you let yourself think that that's the whole picture, you are forgetting how complex people are.

14. *Stick with one feeling at a time.* You will have much more opportunity to learn new behavior if you immediately express yourself rather than trying to put things into perspective. You can make time for that after you have said what you feel like saying. A good way to keep yourself from facing anything is to constantly stifle your expression of one sort of feeling because you are in a hurry to cancel it out with acknowledgment of a contrary feeling. You may have mixed emotions about an issue, but if you want to fully face that issue, try to stick with those feelings one at a time.

15. *Avoid advising, interpreting, and questioning.* As you listen to others in the group, you will often be tempted to offer advice. People can easily be inundated by well-meant advice. They are likely to withdraw, and you are likely to forget that you are in the group to express yourself. Your contribution will be much better received if it consists not of giving advice but of expressing feelings and experiences of your own that the person stimulated. Similarly, when everyone starts taking on the role of the group leader in

providing interpretations, the person speaking is likely to feel that he or she is the only one working and become defensive. People also tend to be defensive when faced with an onslaught of questions. Questions can be asked in ways that open people up rather than closing them down. If you feel inclined to ask a question, experiment with prefacing your question with a declaration of why you have an interest in hearing someone's answer. Let others know of your personal investment in your questions. You will carry your work further if you tell them your personal reactions to the issue rather than questioning them about theirs.

16. *Don't "gossip."* Here gossiping means talking about someone in the third person. Even if the person is not in the room, you get closer to what you want to say if you use "you" rather than "he" or "she." Your group leader may encourage you to pretend that the person you want to talk about is in the room and have you speak directly to this person. Although this exercise may seem artificial at times, it usually leads to a powerful expression of feelings or thoughts. If you doubt this result, watch how the exercise works with others in your group. Or think of someone toward whom you feel anger and see whether you can experience the difference by first saying aloud "I'm angry with him because . . ." and then saying "I'm angry with *you* because . . . "

17. *Don't "Band-Aid."* If you rush in to support or comfort fellow members who are expressing pain, you are not respecting their ability and desire to fully express what they want to say. You probably know from your own experience how good it can feel to get something out instead of having it cut off by someone's ill-timed helpfulness. People grow from living through their pain, so let them do it. Certainly, interactions in a group leave plenty of room for words and gestures of comfort or consolation, but wait until people have gotten through their pain. Otherwise your message is that they always need a "mother" to help them.

18. *Give feedback.* When people express something that touches you, let them know by emphasizing your own feelings and reactions. Even if your feedback is not easy to express and may be difficult to listen to, it can be useful if it is delivered in a caring and concerned manner. In the long run, your willingness to directly and honestly confront another member with your reactions enhances the level of trust within the group and leads you to greater honesty in your daily life. In providing others with feedback, steer clear of telling them what they should do or how they are. Avoid giving quick reassurance or offering them pat solutions for their problems. Rather than telling them how to solve their problems, tell them about your own struggle with your own problems. Emphasize feedback that will give others a clearer sense of how their behavior affects you personally. Avoid judging people, but do let them know what specific behaviors of theirs might be getting in your way in dealing with them. Also, let them know of behaviors that might bring you closer to them.

19. *Avoid storytelling.* If you go on at length to provide others with information about you, you wind up distracting yourself and everyone else. Avoid

narratives of your history. Express what is present, or express what is past if you are struggling with this past event.

20. *Exaggerate.* You can sometimes worry too much about whether you are acting when you focus on a feeling you have. Rather than wondering whether you are exaggerating your emotions, give yourself permission to nurture them a bit and discover where they lead. Of course, you won't want to fake it, but you may get in touch with something genuine by throwing yourself into what you feel.

21. *Be open to feedback.* When others give you feedback about their reactions to your work, remember that, like you, they are there to try out new ways of expressing themselves directly. It is easy to accept their feedback as gospel or to be too quick to reject their insights by rebutting them or explaining away what they say. The most constructive approach is usually to listen and to think their reactions over until you get a grasp on what parts of it fit.

22. *Avoid sarcasm and indirect hostility.* A main goal of participants in an experiential group is to learn to express feelings, including anger, in a direct manner. If you feel angry, say so directly. Do not use pot shots and sarcasm, which people often don't know how to interpret. If you are hostile, which is indirect anger, it not only negatively affects others around you but also builds up inside of you like venom and sickens you. If you learn to express even minor irritations, there is a reduced risk that you will store up negative reactions that are unexpressed, which eventually lead to hostility and are expressed through sarcasm.

23. *React to group leaders.* It's normal for members to react to group leaders with feelings borrowed from the past, from fantasy, and from reality. You can turn this reaction to advantage by making it a special point to explore and express your feelings about your group leaders. Let them know how what they are saying and doing affects you.

24. *Beware of labels.* Watch out for the generalizations, summary statements, and labels you use to describe yourself. For example, you may define yourself as a "loner" and an "outsider," and you may communicate through your behavior that you want people to stay away. Such behavior and self-imposed labels invite others to treat you as an outsider and insist on pigeonholing you for the duration of the group. Be ready to call others if you think they are reducing you to one dimension. And try to guard against assuming that once members have given themselves labels, you are entitled to suppose forever that you've got them figured out.

25. *Make friends with your defenses.* Your defenses may have helped you get where you are today. But they may need modification if you are to make significant changes. Come to respect your defenses by understanding the purpose they serve. You probably already have some idea of how you might sabotage your own work in a group—by rationalizing, withdrawing, denying, or turning a specific criticism into a global "I'm no good." When you become aware of your typical patterns of avoidance, challenge these defenses and try to substitute direct and effective behavior.

26. *Decide for yourself how much to disclose.* To find out about yourself, you need to take some risks by saying more than you are comfortable saying. However, pushing yourself should be distinguished from disclosing things about yourself simply because others seem to expect or need it. If you find that it is difficult for you to share yourself personally in your group, begin by letting others know what makes it hard for you to let yourself be known.

27. *Carry your work outside the group.* You will be finding new ways of expressing yourself within the group. Don't let it go at that! Try these behaviors out in your everyday life with due respect for timing and with caution. On the other hand, don't burden yourself with the expectation that you should express everything that you say in a group situation to a significant person in your life on the outside. For instance, you may role-play with your "father" in a group and discharge feelings of hurt and anger that you have never shared with him. If you value improving your relationship with him, it is not wise to say everything that you released and worked through in a symbolic way in therapy. Instead, decide what you'd most want to say to him, especially what you'd like to tell him about yourself. Be willing to set action-oriented homework assignments for yourself and make a commitment to yourself and your group to follow through with your plans. If through the work you do in a group you become aware that you want a closer relationship and would like to spend more time with him, challenge yourself to carry out behavioral assignments that will help you get what you say you want. Remember, if you want to change, it will be necessary to work and practice outside of the group.

28. *Don't be stopped by setbacks.* You may have a specific vision of how you'd like to behave differently. In spite of formulating specific plans and making a commitment to accomplish your plans, however, you will have relapses at times. Instead of getting discouraged and convincing yourself that you'll never change, be patient with temporary regressions. Realize that you have spent years developing your present patterns. When you are under pressure, you may revert to these old and familiar styles, even though they may not serve you well any longer. Making the changes that you want is often a slow and tedious process.

29. *Express all of your feelings.* Some feelings are easier to express than others. Groups generally focus on those feelings that are causing members some difficulty. Because we usually don't get a chance to explore ways in which our feelings affect us, try to push yourself to talk about those feelings that you frequently try to deny. But you needn't conclude that there is an unspoken rule in the group that limits you to speaking only of problems and conflicts. Share your joys too!

30. *Think about your thinking.* Learn to monitor your self-talk. Identify those beliefs that are contributing to your feeling miserable. For example, if you tell yourself that others could not possibly like you or want a friendship with you once they really got to know you, reflect on how you can easily be setting yourself up for defeat. You may be creating a host of self-fulfilling

prophecies that keep you from feeling and acting the way you'd like. Once you have identified some patterns of negative thinking, bring them to a session, and begin to challenge them. You can learn how to argue with those voices in your head that keep you from becoming the person you want to be.

31. *Take responsibility for what you accomplish.* The leaders and members of your group will no doubt be interested in drawing you out, but remember that in the last analysis what you accomplish in the group is up to you. Don't wait for others to call on you. Learn to ask for what you want. You will determine what and how much you get.

32. *Be familiar with your culture.* Recognize that your cultural background does influence who you are. Discover the ways in which you continue to be affected by your cultural environment. Although you can appreciate values that you have gotten from your culture, be open to questioning the degree to which you might want to modify some of them. You can ask yourself whether certain ways of living are still in your best interest. If you decide that some behaviors are no longer effective, use the group to think of ways to make the changes you desire.

33. *Respect confidentiality.* Keep in mind how easy it might be to inadvertently betray the confidences of others. Make it a practice not to talk about what others are doing in your group or what they are experiencing. If you choose to talk about the group to others, talk about yourself and what you are learning. If at any time you become unsure that confidentiality is being respected, bring this matter up in the group. If you do not feel trusting because you are afraid that others will talk, this doubt will surely hamper your participation.

34. *Develop a reading program.* Reading can be therapeutic and can also provide you with material to bring up in your therapy. Select books that will help you put your life experiences in a new perspective or books that can teach you new patterns of thinking and behaving.

35. *Write in your journal.* If you hope to rely on memory alone to sort through all that you experience in your group, you'll probably find that much of what you did and observed will be lost. Even brief entries in a journal can be most useful in helping you monitor yourself and keep track of how well you are attaining your goals.

•   •   •   •   •   •   •   •   •   •   •   •   •   •   •   •   •   •   •

Depending on the type of group you are leading and the nature of the membership, you can formulate your own written list of suggestions for maximizing the group experience. It helps to have a list that members can keep and review periodically. Some group practitioners might argue that it is better not to provide a list like the one in the box, on the grounds that members should struggle to find their own way. We do not agree. Our experience is that much floundering occurs when members are not given some idea of how best to do the work they came to the group to do. Moreover, we have seen group members who are psychologically wounded by hostility over their questioning, storytelling, and gossiping and who then become defensive and withdrawn for the remainder of the group. We think this outcome is unnecessary and unproductive and that it is not likely to occur if members have been told how best to participate in a group.

Preparing Leaders

In addition to preparing members to get the most from a group, you need to get yourself ready to be fully present in the groups you lead. If you do not devote time to preparing psychologically, the group is likely to suffer. In approaching a new group, for example, you might ask yourself these questions:

- How ready do I feel for this group? Am I feeling available for the members?
- Do I want to do this group? How alive and enthusiastic do I feel?
- How effective am I feeling in my personal life? Am I doing in my life what I hope my members will do in their lives?
- Am I feeling professionally confident?
- Do I believe in the process of a group, or am I doing a group merely because I was told to?

In addition to preparing yourself before meeting a group for the first time, you can use at least some of the following procedures to get ready for an upcoming session:

- Spend some time, if only a few minutes, in relaxation before you go into your group. Take time to reflect on what you'd like to accomplish.
- Be aware of your own thoughts and feelings so that you can use them in your work with others.
- Try for yourself some of the exercises and catalysts you will ask your group to use. Thus, if you intend to ask the members how they are seeing themselves and how they are feeling about themselves, ask yourself these same questions.
- Spend some time, perhaps at lunch or dinner, with your co-leader. If the two of you are not attuned, your work will be disjointed. Talk about how you are feeling about yourselves, about working as a team, about going into the group, and about any of the members. Do you respect each other? Do you trust each other? Is one doing most of the work?
- Devote some time to thinking about the previous session. Where did the group leave off? How can you bridge the gap between the last session and the upcoming one?

Concluding Comments

In this chapter we have discussed preparation as a technique for promoting group effectiveness. We have emphasized screening interviews, preliminary sessions, clarification of goals, suggestions to help members get the most from a group, and ways for leaders to get ready. Many problems in the working stage of a group arise because of inadequate preparation, which results in a lack of clarity about the nature of the group and about how best to participate in it. These problems can be avoided by developing some of your own preparation techniques or using some that we have suggested here.

Questions and Activities

1. Do you agree with our emphasis on preparing group members? Drawing from books listed in our bibliography or other books with which you are familiar, review the reasons that some might give for not preparing members for a group.
2. Suppose you are working in an agency and are asked to organize a group for a particular population. How might you go about it? Discuss such matters as recruiting, screening, selecting, and preparing members. What would you say to prospective members about what you expect of them and what they should expect of you?
3. How might you set up a long-term group differently from a short-term group? Would there be any differences in how you designed an open group (one with changing membership) and a closed group (one with the same members)?
4. What is your position regarding screening of members? What specific factors would you look for in deciding to include or exclude someone? How might you tell someone you did not want him or her in a group? Would you provide alternatives? If so, what might these be?
5. At this point in your professional development, what kinds of groups and what kinds of populations do you regard yourself as qualified to lead? What groups might you be most interested in forming and leading?
6. What are some advantages of pregroup preparation for members? What specific information would you give members before the initial group meeting? How might you go about orienting them?
7. We discuss the advantages of preliminary sessions. Can you think of any disadvantages or potential hazards of such sessions?
8. Suppose a member is concerned at a preliminary meeting about whether what goes on in the group will stay there. What would you say? Would you open up the topic of confidentiality for group discussion, or declare your own rules?
9. Under what circumstances, if any, would you breach the confidentiality of your group members' disclosures? How might you explain this exception in the screening interview or the first meeting?
10. Assume that an adolescent asks you whether you would tell her parents about something she said in the group. How would you respond?
11. Think of a group that you would be interested in designing. Write a brief proposal for this group with a specific target population, and present the proposal to your class. Others in the class can give you feedback on your presentation as well as on the proposal itself.

12. Break into dyads, with one person assuming the role of a candidate for a group and the other conducting a screening interview. After about ten minutes, switch roles. Or break into triads, with the third person giving feedback. Partners should discuss how it feels to be the group leader doing the interviewing as well as the prospective participant being interviewed.

13. Write a list of group rules that you might distribute or at least discuss with a group. Present these rules to a small group of classmates to get their reactions to your policies and to consider rules included in their lists but not in yours.

14. We make several suggestions for orienting and preparing participants for a group experience. Which of these suggestions are you inclined to accept, and which do you reject? Discuss.

15. You are meeting your group for the first time, and a member asks how he can get the most from this group. How might you respond?

16. Do you think it is important for members to clarify their goals before entering a group? Explain. What would you do, or not do, to promote this clarification?

17. Some group leaders use written contracts that outline their expectations of members and what members can expect of them. What advantages and disadvantages do you see in this procedure? With what kind of group(s) might you use written contracts?

18. You discover that several members are talking outside the group about matters discussed in the group. What might you do?

19. What are your views about asking members to do reading or writing? If you see value in such exercises, how might you present them to your group? What would you hope the members would gain? How would your answers to these questions vary with the population of the group?

20. Can you overprepare members for a group? How? What effect might over-preparation have on the group process?

21. We mention the need for co-leaders to attune themselves. What are the signs and consequences of a lack of preparation?

22. Discuss your reactions to any part or all of the box "Guidelines and Suggestions for Group Members."

23. We suggest writing autobiographies as a technique to get members focused for a group. Write your own brief autobiography, mentioning critical turning points in your life and the effect they have had on you. If you are reading this book as part of a class, you may want to share with your classmates what this experience was like for you.

24. Another focusing technique we describe is to ask members to imagine they are a book. Do this exercise yourself. Again, you might want to form small groups and share this "book of you."

25. In this chapter we talk about the use of structure in groups. What are your thoughts about the balance between too much structure and not enough structure? What problems do you see with either of these extremes? Which side might you be inclined toward? Discuss.

CHAPTER FOUR

Techniques for the Initial Stage

$\mathbf{I}$f a leader has done a good job in the preparation phase of a group, members are likely to come to the first session with a focus and a readiness to work that will help them during the initial stage. This stage is critical because the group's identity is being formed. In this chapter we discuss some of the basic characteristics of a group during this first stage, and we provide some techniques for getting the group started and for dealing with initial resistance.

Characteristics of the Initial Stage

At the first session, both the members and the leaders are usually anxious. The leaders may wonder what the group will be like, whether they will be able to deal effectively with what comes up, and whether they will be able to bring a group of strangers together in such a way that the trust necessary for effective work is created.

Members are typically anxious about being rejected, about revealing themselves, about meeting new people, and about being in a new situation. These general fears of members are mixed with anxiety about the specific issues they intend to explore and about whether they will be able to do so. They are not quite certain about what to expect in a group, which heightens their concerns about fitting in and being accepted. They are apt to worry about whether they will be on the inside or the outside of the group. Members may also be resistant, especially if the group is not a voluntary one. They may be there physically but not psychologically, they may be skeptical about the value of groups or the purpose of the group, or they may wonder how the group will be of use to them.

Even if members want to be in the group, they may be unaware of how to get involved. Should they wait to be invited to speak? What should they talk about? How personal should they be? How much detail should they give? How can they use the group to understand and deal with their problems? Should they behave in the group just as they do in everyday life, or should they act differently?

Trust is a basic consideration during the early stage of a group. Members may ask themselves: "Is it safe for me to be myself?" "Will what I say be listened to?" "Can I risk revealing parts of myself that I generally keep hidden?" "What will people think of me if I reveal what I'm really like?" "Do I dare share my reactions to other members of the group?" "If I'm having negative feelings about being in the group, is it appropriate to reveal these feelings openly?" "And if I do, what kind of reaction will I get from the others?"

Members are also usually concerned about outcomes. They wonder whether they will be better off after taking part. Will the group make a difference to them, or will it be a waste of time? Will they find out that they are "crazy" or that there is something about themselves that they cannot stand?

Finally, during the initial stage, people are developing roles within the group, forming power structures and alliances, carving out identities, testing the leader and other members, deciding whether they are being included in or excluded from the group, attempting to please the leader, and attempting to meet the expectations of other members.

Physical Arrangements and Settings

An important initial responsibility of the leader is to decide where the group will be held and to arrange this setting in a way that is conducive to group work. Two important considerations are privacy and freedom from distractions. Sometimes, for example, group leaders think that meeting outdoors is appealing in good weather because of the informality, but such a setting generally lacks privacy and is a source of distractions.

Because the physical setting contributes to the climate of a group, some degree of attractiveness is necessary. If the meeting place has no windows and is poorly ventilated, if it is cold, or if it is uncomfortable, attention is bound to be drawn away from exploring personal issues. In a clinical setting or the ward of an institution, the walls are usually bare, and the group room may be sterile and uninviting. The leader can encourage members to think of some imaginative ways of brightening the atmosphere. This technique helps the members assume some responsibility.

Seating arrangements are important. A group that meets in a room where members are physically separated by tables or otherwise spread out has a different quality from a group that meets in a setting that promotes eye contact and allows for some closeness. When a member cannot see all the other members, when some members are in corners of the room, when some are sitting behind others, and when other physical barriers are present, psychological distance and fragmentation can be expected. By the same token, when members are too crowded together, closeness is forced on them. Another consideration is that an atmosphere that is too comfortable and informal can foster inattentiveness. At times group leaders want to get rid of uncomfortable chairs. Mattresses and large, overstuffed bean bags, however, may invite a prone posture that causes members to tune out of the session and perhaps even be lulled to sleep.

Although the considerations pertaining to physical arrangements may seem obvious, leaders can easily overlook such matters. We encourage you to experiment with physical arrangements to see whether they make a difference in what goes on in a group.

In the sections that follow we discuss techniques for getting groups started. In using these catalysts, you might listen for the themes mentioned in the earlier section on characteristics of the initial stage and use them as clues in deciding how to proceed.

Techniques for Getting Acquainted

Introductions are one of the first items of business. Depending on the type of group, a variety of approaches can be tried. Also, whether the group is an open one or a closed one determines some of the techniques that are best used in helping members get acquainted. In a group where members come and go, obviously, it is crucial that new members be introduced as they enter.

Learning names.   One technique is to have people introduce themselves by name and say anything about themselves they would like the group to know. Before members start, they are asked to repeat the names of all those who have introduced themselves previously. Our preference is to avoid going around mechanically in a circle. We encourage the members to bring themselves into the group without being called upon by us. We prefer to let members spontaneously enter the group by their own choice, for this process gives us some information about them. In this way members can learn one another's names in a few minutes by sheer repetition. This practice also keeps the process of getting acquainted moving quickly, as members are anxious to speak up before the list of names to be remembered gets too long.

Introducing oneself.   Leaders can ask members to introduce themselves in different ways. For example, they might introduce themselves as the people they'd like to be at the time of their final session. This technique gets people to think about their goals. It gives others a sense of what each person hopes for from the group, and it gives all a chance to begin risking themselves. Or leaders can ask members to make a conscious effort to say something about themselves that is risky and difficult. This technique provides a way for members to decide at the outset how much they are willing to risk in the group.

The following list gives a few examples of other catalysts that leaders can use to help members begin to get acquainted:

- "Could each of you make a brief statement about how it was for you to come to this first session today? What did you think about before coming here? What were you feeling? And what are you thinking and feeling now?"
- "What do you expect this group to be like for you? What do you hope it will be like? What do you fear it will be like?"
- "Let's have each of you say how you found out about this group. What were you told about the group?"
- "What do you most hope you'll learn in this group? What are you willing to do to get what you want?"
- "Who knows anyone else in this group? Would you state any prior relationships any of you have?"
- "What are your greatest fears, if you have any, about being in this group?"
- "Did you want to come to this group? If so, what motivated you? If you didn't want to come here, how was it for you to be 'sent' here? Now that you're here, how is it for you?"
- "What previous experience have you had in counseling or in groups? What have you gotten from any of the groups you've been in before?"
- "Who has a vested interest in your being here?"

- "What do you want from this group for the next 12 weeks that we'll be together?"
- "What in your lives are you struggling with at this time?"

Introducing someone else. Another technique for getting people introduced consists of asking members to pair up and get to know as much as possible about their partner so that they can later introduce the partner to the entire group. Partners should avoid bombarding each other with probing questions. They can instead be active listeners and can share as much about themselves as they choose to. This technique gives members practice in speaking about themselves to one other person. The exercise typically takes about 20 minutes. The leader can announce when the time is half up so that partners can exchange the roles of listener and speaker. Otherwise, quiet people may spend the entire 20 minutes in polite listening and say only a few words about themselves. Before the reverse introductions begin, members can tell their partners what, if anything, they do not want the group to know. As a variation, instead of introducing each other, members can say what it was like for them to listen to their partner. If this is done, however, it is important that members avoid putting the focus on their partner or telling specific details about the partner. Instead, what is important is that members tell how *they* were affected.

Setting a time limit. You can give members an egg timer and ask them to relate the aspects of themselves that they deem significant in not more than three minutes. Members can share something of their past, focus on their current lives, or express their hopes for their future. They can also share whatever they are feeling at the moment. This is a good follow-up technique to the previous one, because it gives each member an opportunity for self-presentation. You can begin this process yourself in order to teach the members, through modeling, how to talk about themselves. It is best that members not react or respond during this go-around. Discussion can follow after everyone has had a turn. Anyone with strong reservations about taking part in the exercise can simply pass the timer to another person. It is good practice for you not to focus on this person at this time and interrupt the flow of the go-around.

This technique will often provide you with ideas for later use. You can note especially how members use their allotted time. Some run over in an attempt to convey much detail about themselves, whereas others quickly run out of things to say and are embarrassed.

Using dyads and small groups. To lessen members' feelings of being intimidated by a large group, you can ask them to form dyads or triads for about ten minutes and get acquainted with their partners. Then, they can find new partners for another ten minutes. Depending on the size of the group and the people in it, switches can be made between two and ten times. Or, after a number of changes, a dyad or triad can join with another dyad or triad and continue the exercise. This technique gives most of the participants at least a brief opportunity to make some contact with others and to say something about themselves. The use of various combinations of small groups is an excellent icebreaker and a good way to begin to generate trust and interaction within the group. Eventually, you can convene the entire group and ask members to share briefly what they experienced in the small groups.

How much structure should these small groups be given? Generally, we favor bringing some focus to these subgroups, even though we allow them to deviate from discussing the questions suggested. The advantage of encouraging discussion of particular issues is that the entire group can later focus on certain themes. Any of the questions we suggested in the section on introducing oneself would be appropriate here.

The use of subgroups entails the risk of fostering permanent alliances. Therefore, you might check to be sure that the membership of subgroups changes frequently. If alliances do form within the group, you might comment on this development.

The leader's role. Leaders should keep things moving in the initial go-arounds when people are introducing themselves, for in this way everyone has several opportunities to make statements, and there is no sustained focus on a single individual. Leaders should also discourage members from asking questions, especially about why people feel as they do. If a question-and-answer format is established at the beginning, it can continue for the whole course of the group. To keep the focus moving from person to person, leaders often find it useful to have a number of go-arounds, asking several of the questions we suggested. Asking only one question at a time lessens the chances that members will feel overwhelmed.

Leaders can be actively involved in the introduction process in order to begin to establish trust. They can share their feelings about starting the group, can say what they expect and hope for, can tell something about their experience in leading groups, and, depending on the particular group, can disclose something about themselves personally. They can add what they gain from leading groups and what they hope to learn or experience in this group. Remarks about what they are aware of at the moment are often the most valuable, because such disclosures model a focus on the sharing of present experiences for the members.

Techniques for Focusing Members

Paying attention to the group process. As a group is starting to take shape, it is important for leaders to pay attention to the subtle aspects of the emerging group process and to teach members how to recognize their own reactions. At the first session we sometimes ask members to quietly size up everyone in the room. We encourage them to silently focus on their assumptions, reactions, and perceptions regarding each individual. We always stress that we will not ask them to reveal these reactions at this time. Our purpose is to assist the members in clarifying some of the thoughts and feelings they have as they are put into a new group of people.

During the initial stage we make a concerted effort to teach members how to pay attention to their own behavior in the context of what is occurring in the session. At the first session we frequently ask "Whom are you most comfortable with in this group, and why?" Then again, at the third meeting, we might ask "Whom are you most uncomfortable with, and why?" We encourage members to become aware of the particular individuals whom they most remember or whom they think about outside of the session.

As members are making themselves known through the process of "checking in," or saying at the beginning of a group what they want out of it, we silently take note of their style of speech and their use of metaphors. For example, members sometimes use vivid language that conveys some of their underlying feelings and beliefs. Samples of some of these loaded phrases are: "My fear is that I'll be fried and grilled in this group." "I've heard about these groups where people are expected to spill their guts." "If I open up, people might pounce on me." "There have been times when I've made myself vulnerable and people blasted me." As the group is just beginning to evolve, we rarely interpret the members' use of language; rather, we take note of it and look for patterns and connections if they continue to develop over time.

At the second meeting of a group, we often begin by asking each member to check in by addressing some of the following questions: "Whom were you aware of as you were going home last week?" "Whom were you thinking of and what were you thinking about as you were coming to the group this morning?" "What most stood out for you about your experience in the group last week?" "Did you have any reactions about our first meeting during this past week?" Our basic purpose in presenting this line of questions is to teach members the importance of paying attention to the ways in which they are affected when they are in the group and to underscore the importance of expressing persistent thoughts and feelings. During the initial phase we frequently remind participants how important it is that they not keep their reactions to themselves. We tell them that our concern is not with what they *say* but, rather, with what they keep to themselves. For instance, if members are aware that they are frightened of speaking out because they are intimidated by the group leaders, it is imperative that they let this fear be known.

Focusing on issues outside the group. We have indicated the emphasis that we put on harnessing the group's energy in focusing on the here-and-now interactions within the room. We think that paying attention to how one behaves in the group situation tells a good deal about one's behavior outside of the group. Indeed, we find that if we are successful in getting members to deal with their here-and-now experience of being in a new group, it frequently leads them to reveal the pressing concerns in their daily life that brought them to the group in the first place. Yet we also employ techniques that assist members in focusing on issues outside the group. Our techniques have the general purpose of enabling members to talk more concretely about themselves and less about other people in their lives. If they do talk about others, we encourage them to say how they are affected rather than merely giving detailed stories about others. We employ various open-ended questions to get members focused on outside issues that they want to explore in their group:

- "If your life were frozen now, how would that be?"
- "If this were your last opportunity for therapy, what would you pick to work on?"
- "Whom in your life are you concerned about now?"
- "What stops you from being the person who you say you want to be?"
- "What do you most hope that you will get from this group?"
- "What are some specific thoughts or beliefs that tend to interfere with your functioning as effectively as you might like?"
- "What are some feelings that are a source of concern to you?"
- "If there were just a few specific behaviors that you could modify, what would they be?"

Techniques for Creating Trust

There is no single technique or even a set of techniques that alone creates trust. As we emphasized in Chapter 1, you, as the leader, are your most important technique. The kind of person you are and your ability to establish direct contact with others are likely to be major determinants of the level of trust in your groups. Using techniques without first establishing a good relationship with group members is likely to result in suspicion and holding back on the part of the members. Such a relationship is best established by paying attention to the needs of individual members, responding to them in respectful ways, appropriately self-disclosing, being willing to state your expectations openly, encouraging members to talk directly to one another and doing so yourself, being sensitive to the fears and anxieties of the members, and providing people with opportunities to openly say whatever they are feeling or thinking.

In the initial stage a basic task of a group is dealing with mistrust. Mistrust takes several forms. Members can mistrust themselves. They may ask themselves: "Do I trust myself enough to look at what is going on in my life?" "Am I trusting enough to express my feelings?" "Am I afraid that if I begin to feel sad or angry, I'll feel that way forever?" Members can also mistrust other members. They may have negative reactions to some members that contribute to their hesitation in making themselves known. Finally, members can mistrust the leader or co-leaders. Although some participants may naively have an automatic sense of confidence and trust in group leaders, others may have initial reactions of mistrust and cynicism because they perceive leaders as authority figures—mothers, fathers, police officers.

The issue of trust is never settled once and for all. The issue is especially pressing during the initial stage, but it continues to manifest itself in different forms throughout the time the group is together. We tell members that their trust may rise and fall. Furthermore, we don't think it is necessarily a bad sign if group trust diminishes. What is essential, however, is that the members demonstrate a willingness to acknowledge their lag in trust. Members need to learn that the more threatening the material explored becomes, the more the issue of trust is central. Certainly the delicate nature of trust is a focal point for the early stage. We continually let members know that trust is not something that merely happens to them; rather, it is the outcome of the risky steps they are willing to take to bring this level of safety into their group. We emphasize that a good place to begin is by talking about what makes it difficult for them to feel a sense of trust in one another.

The leader's most important task in dealing with mistrust is to give people many opportunities to talk about their feelings early in the group. If work is to proceed, mistrust must be first recognized and then dealt with in the group. If it is not, a hidden agenda develops, the lack of trust is expressed in indirect ways, and the group grinds to a halt. If a basic sense of trust is not established at the outset and the group leader tries to push an agenda too soon, serious problems can be predicted: lack of enthusiasm, little energy, and awkward silences.

Consider the following example of how a hidden agenda during an early session can temporarily inhibit the trust level in the group. The previous week one member, George, experienced a catharsis, and many members seemed emotionally involved in his work. On returning, however, people seemed more guarded than they had been the week before, and there was a mood of quietness in the group. With the prodding of the group leader, members eventually revealed what was behind their hesitation to speak up. Some were frightened at how quickly George had let go of deep feelings. They were not sure what they should do about the reactions they had. Some did not want to interrupt his work, but they were very aware of being deeply touched by him. Some who were moved personally were afraid to acknowledge this for fear that they might "lose control" as George had. Although some members wanted to get involved by discussing their own problems, they put the brakes on themselves for fear that they would be inappropriately interrupting what he was doing. Other members were angry because they felt that he had been "left hanging." They couldn't see what good it had done for him to get so worked up and then not get an answer to his problem.

Still other clients finally confessed that they were burdening themselves with "performance standards." They thought that to be accepted in the group, they would have to display a great deal of emotional intensity. They were afraid that if they did not cry, others might perceive them as being superficial and "out of it." The point we wish to make is that all of these reactions are fertile material for highly productive interaction *if* the members are indeed willing to bring them up. By fully expressing and exploring such reactions, members genuinely develop the basis of trust. On the other hand, if members "sit on" their reactions, the group loses its vitality. We often say that those group issues that do not get talked about almost always develop into a hidden agenda that constipates the individuals and the group.

You can recognize when a climate of trust has been created because members then express their reactions without fear of censure and being judged, are actively involved in the activities in the group, make themselves known to others in personal ways, take risks both in the group and in everyday life, focus on themselves and not on others, actively work in the group on meaningful personal issues, disclose persistent feelings of lack of trust, and both support and challenge others in the group.

By contrast, there are some clear signs when trust is lacking. Some of these indications of a low level of trust include:

- Participants are unwilling to initiate work.
- They are unwilling to contribute when they are called on for their reactions.
- They keep negative feelings to themselves, share them only with a clique, or express them in indirect ways.
- Members take refuge in long-winded storytelling.
- Participants hide behind intellectualizations.
- They are deliberately vague and focus endlessly on others instead of on themselves.
- They are excessively quiet.
- Participants put more energy into "helping" others or giving others advice than into sharing their personal concerns.
- Some maintain that they do not have any problems that the group can help them with.
- Others are unwilling to deal openly with conflict or even to acknowledge the existence of conflict.
- Some exert an excessive degree of group pressure as a way of achieving conformity to norms.

When trust is lacking, members sometimes make judgmental statements, which have the effect of inhibiting open participation. For instance, a member may say to another person: "You're acting! You never talk about yourself. You're always judging everyone else." Or another member may express a feeling of being judged by asserting: "If I don't say it just the right way, I get jumped on. Everyone attacks in here. I don't know what I'm doing in this group."

So far we have stressed the components of building trust that cannot be replaced by exercises alone. We have emphasized paying attention to the relationship that the leader is developing with members and that the members are developing with one another. Once members have been encouraged to express their lack of trust, the building of trust can be encouraged by using techniques that foster a sense of community. We present here a few techniques that facilitate the process of establishing trust and security within a group.

Identifying fears. The anxieties that participants have about themselves, other members, and the leader or co-leaders can be fruitfully explored as one way to generate trust. If these fears are kept secret, they are simply magnified and continue to grow. If they are acknowledged openly, they subside or at least do not inhibit participation in the group.

To help participants explore their fears, the leader can ask them to close their eyes and imagine the worst thing that could happen to them in the group. Henry, for example, sees himself being verbally attacked by all the women in the group. Because he doesn't know how to respond, he imagines himself becoming paralyzed and crying unceasingly. After the exercise, members can share how they felt about their fantasy. If they like, they can share the fantasy and the fear itself. This technique allows members to express their fears openly instead of letting them fester inside unacknowledged. We find over and over that what causes problems in a group is not the feelings and thoughts people *do* express but those reactions that they do *not* express.

Dealing with fears. As a leader you have a number of ways of working with fears once they have been identified. Let's suppose that Jill says "I'm afraid of being myself in here, because people will reject me." She can live out this fantasy in the group by imagining each person systematically rejecting her. She can also imagine herself leaving and having the worst feelings possible. After imagining these scenes, Jill can be asked to make the rounds and say out loud, in a few words, what she guesses each person might say to her. This method allows her to face some of her fears by exaggerating them and imagining the worst possible outcomes. Another approach is simply to let her talk about her fear of rejection in the group. She may admit that she has this fear in most social situations and so avoids new situations lest she be rejected. Another technique is to have all those in the group who share Jill's fear form an inner circle. She can lead the group by encouraging them to talk about the ways in which they are similar to her and about how they deal with their fear of being rejected.

Another way to deal with mistrust is to ask participants to imagine what it would take for them to feel secure enough to reveal themselves in significant ways. Some may say that they would want to know that they were not alone in what they felt; others may say that they would want some assurance that they wouldn't be attacked by others; still others may add that they would need a group of people who cared and were supportive. Members can also break into subgroups to discuss what inhibits their willingness to trust. Then, when the whole group reconvenes, you can ask what characteristics the group needs if a trusting climate is to come about. Giving participants time to imagine ideal circumstances in these ways builds trust.

Another trust-building exercise after people have been together for at least a couple of sessions and have had some opportunity to formulate some impressions of one another is to ask them to look at each of the others in turn and ask themselves: "How is it to be in the group with this person? Am I willing to be open with this person?" Or participants can ask themselves: "Whom in this group do I feel the closest to? Whom do I feel the most distant from? Whom would it be easiest and hardest for me to get to know?" After a few minutes, you can ask whether anyone is willing to report any reactions. This device brings out into the open reservations that participants might have, and it can facilitate a discussion of how members are being affected by one another. If members are having doubts or reservations about others, these reactions need to be acknowledged and openly dealt with if trust is to be established.

Physical trust-building exercises have a different flavor from the techniques we have been advocating. For example, in the blind-trust walk a member is blindfolded and led by another. This exercise forces the "blind" individuals to trust their guides to keep them from stumbling. They can find it exhilarating to relinquish control and have confidence in another.

Although physical exercises can be worthwhile, we rarely use them, for they can produce a short-lived exhilaration and can deflect people from talking about their concerns regarding trust. In our view, trust develops slowly or not at all if the leader uses mechanical techniques rather than facilitating the group's own struggle toward earned trust. The use of structured exercises tends to focus people on variables outside of themselves. Our preference is to facilitate trust not by using interactional exercises but by encouraging clients to express what is going on within them. Doing so challenges them to honestly share their fears and resistances.

Techniques for Dealing with Initial Resistance

One of the best ways of developing trust is to recognize the beginning signs of resistance within a group and to deal with them. Leaders should have respect for resistance as a natural part of the group process. Regardless of how highly motivated clients may be to get involved in their group, awkwardness and tentativeness permeate the atmosphere until people begin to get a sense of one another. As a group is forming, we expect participants to have reservations in revealing aspects of themselves that they generally do not freely share with strangers. They have good reason to feel threatened, for the unknown does not inspire a sense of security. Resistance is not simply lack of cooperation, and not all resistance is negative. After all, it is to some extent healthy to be cautious about making oneself known until it seems safe to do so. Thus, resistance is not something to be avoided or bypassed. Pretending that resistance does not exist will not make it disappear. Ignoring both obvious and subtle signs of resistance leads only to a group's becoming bogged down. Blaming the members for being stubborn and unmotivated is likely to increase their defensiveness. Blaming yourself for your ineptness as a group leader does not help. Resistance can be constructively explored only by encouraging participants to state some of the factors that are keeping them from getting involved and by acknowledging these sources of their resistance.

Being sensitive to fears. An obvious source of resistance in the initial stage of a group is pushing participants too quickly to overcome the fears and anxieties that are normal at this stage. These fears can be compounded if a member volunteers extremely emotional and traumatic material early in the group's history. Leaders should be sensitive to this possibility. Instead of being hungry for drama, they should patiently explore the here-and-now fears and resistances that are an inevitable part of a new group.

Modeling. A good technique for overcoming resistance in the initial stage is modeling by the leader. When you are experiencing resistance from members, you can give your reactions without blaming them. If there are many silences during an early session, for instance, you might say any of the following:

- "What makes it difficult to talk in here?"
- "The silence is difficult for me. I wonder how it is for others in here."
- "Some of you are saying that you feel a sense of closeness with others in this group. I am having trouble trusting this closeness that you say you have with one another. It seems to me that some important things are not being said in here."

You can share how you experience the resistance and how you are affected by it, and you can invite members to say what they are experiencing. Such modeling encourages members to express their feelings and is an important and direct way of dealing with any resistance that is brewing in a group.

Working with involuntary groups. Resistance can be a special problem in groups composed of involuntary clients. Here we briefly discuss resistance as a characteristic of clients who are required to attend a group, and we describe some techniques for dealing with this resistance in a therapeutic fashion. Too often leaders assume that not much will occur in involuntary groups because members are forced to attend. This attitude is easily communicated to and picked up by the members. The opportunities for significant change in such groups should not be overlooked.

In general, people who come to a group as a condition of parole, as a part of treatment on the ward in a mental-health facility, or on the order of a judge are somewhat closed. They probably haven't been told much about how groups function or about what they might gain from participating. Thus, they have a cynical, show-me attitude and a passive style of resisting; they say little and expect to be questioned. Such members may have some of the following thoughts and feelings:

- "I'll say as little as possible, and that way I won't give anyone any ammunition to use against me."
- "They might be able to get my body here to this group, but I'll be damned if they'll get anything out of me."
- "Why should I open up and trust these leaders? They've never been in my shoes. How could they possibly understand me?"
- "I can't see why I should let anyone in here know what I'm thinking. I've survived by being tough all my life. Why should I start to trust people now, and why should I begin to need anybody for anything?"
- "This is just another game. I'll figure out the rules of the game, say the right thing, and then maybe I'll get out quicker."
- "My big problem is that I got caught. I'll be careful from now on and just not get caught."
- "These guys leading the group are supposed to be experts, so I'll let them show me. I'll sit back and watch and make them prove themselves to me. I'll show them that whatever they have to offer won't work."

If resistant members are encouraged to verbalize these thoughts, the words they use can provide material for inventing a technique to explore the resistance further. For example, the client who uses the word *ammunition* can fantasize out loud about what other group members might "shoot" her with. The person who says that nothing will be gotten out of him may be asked to pretend that each of the other members of the group is trying to break into him, as if he were a strongbox with treasures inside, and he can then specify what each person is going to try to do to get inside him. The person who thinks the leaders have never been in her shoes can be asked to talk about what she sees in the leaders that convinces her that they will not be able to share her experiences. The person who says that talk never changes anything can be asked to identify some things that matter to him that talk is not going to change. The point is that leaders should identify resistance in a group and then work to make it explicit. In doing so they are training the group members to express themselves, and they are helping establish a climate of trust because they are communicating to clients that they understand and respect their resistance and are willing to work with it rather than trying to argue it away. In a subtle way this technique bypasses resistance, because members who came determined not to talk are now talking. Leaders should be careful to present the technique in clear language, with a minimum of jargon.

Another potentially useful device is simply to allow the members to express openly for a time their feelings about being forced into a group, without comment from the leader and especially without the implication that they shouldn't feel that way. This technique is a good one to use at the beginning, because it may be the first time that anyone has listened with respect to what these people have to say, and this respect can be the basis for building trust. Eventually the leader can begin to deal with the feelings of resentment, hostility, helplessness, and defiance by saying "Now that you have expressed these feelings, what can you do about them?" This technique leads the group beyond complaining and prevents the meeting from becoming merely a bitch session. It provides the beginning of contact and the beginning of a group.

Another technique for dealing with resistance in clients who are required to attend a group is to make brief contacts with them individually and to spend some time getting to know them. Clients, especially those who live together and attend the group as a part of a treatment program, frequently have had no orientation. They are merely told to attend. A brief contact or several contacts outside the group can be the beginning of rapport.

A direct technique for use in a session is to encourage questions about how the group will function, what the leader's role will be, and related matters. Some members may assume that whatever they say will be recorded and perhaps used against them. You can help establish trust in this situation by being honest about your role in the group and about how much of what goes on in the session you will report. For example, if you are required to keep notes on clients and put a summary of their progress in a file, you can assure members that you will discuss with them what is going into their folders. Or you can role-play what you are going to say to supervisors about clients.

A basic approach for working with involuntary groups is to inform members that although they must attend the sessions, you are open to suggestions from them, and they will have a significant impact on how the time is used. You can then point out some possibilities. Members who come to a group reluctant to do more than put in their time may find value in attending if alternatives for using that time are explored. Also, members should have an immediate opportunity to evaluate the group. Resistance can often be lessened when members are encouraged to assume some responsibility for how the group functions.

Another freedom sometimes available to involuntary clients is not to participate in a session. They are obliged to be there physically, but they can form an outer circle where participation is not required or allowed. If they change their minds, they can join the inner circle, which is a working group. There may be some limitations to the use of this technique: it may not be allowed by the institution, or the working members in the inner circle may object to being observed by the silent members.

Techniques for Starting a Session

We have talked at length about preparing members and getting a group started, but we also want to give some attention to ways of starting a particular session. When a group is in its initial stage of development, we typically begin each session with at least one go-around. The practice of teaching members to at least briefly check in permits everyone to have some sense of what others are wanting. If we quickly focus on the first person who speaks and do not allow others to check in, we often miss potential themes and ways of linking members with common issues. Leaders may expect that group members will arrive ready to begin work, but it's generally helpful to spend a few minutes getting focused. It is sometimes useful to facilitate connections between sessions, especially with work left unfinished at a previous session. In a typical go-around members declare what they want from this session and whether they wish to discuss anything left over from the last meeting. Leaders may ask people who disclosed important material at the previous session whether they had reactions during the week to their disclosures or have further thoughts about what they did. This technique provides an opportunity for linking sessions and for following up on clients. Let us caution leaders to intervene when members get too detailed in their process of checking in and clarifying how they would like to use time for this session. If leaders do not intervene, it is very possible that most of the session will be consumed by the checking-in exercise. Leaders need to be alert during the initial go-around to avoid interventions that invite people to become emotionally involved. Surely this process of briefly checking in must be sensitively handled, and members often need the leader's guidance in getting to the point.

The following remarks indicate other ways of getting a group focused:

- "What do you most want from today's session?"
- "I'd like to have a go-around in which each person completes the sentence 'Right now I am aware of . . .' "
- "Close your eyes, realize that the next two hours are set aside for you, and ask yourself what you want and what you are willing to do to get it."
- "If your best friend were to introduce you in this group, what would that person be likely to say about you?"
- "Last week we left off with . . ."
- "Do any of you have thoughts about last week's session or any unfinished business from then that you want to bring up now?"
- "What would you most want us to know about you?"
- "How would you like for this session to be different from the previous one?"
- "What are you willing to do to get what you say you want?"
- "Have you thought about anything that you talked about at the last session?"
- "What were you aware of as you were getting ready to come to the group this afternoon?"
- "What fears or doubts do you have about this group, if any?"
- "When you think about this group and how it has been for you, are there any aspects that you would like to change?"
- "If you are in this group now because you were sent here, how do you feel about it?"

Techniques for Ending a Session

During the first few sessions, it is a good idea to spend some time in asking the members to say something about how they view their participation. We discuss issues and techniques for ending sessions in more detail in Chapter 7, but at this point we describe bringing closure to the first few sessions. Questions such as the following are useful catalysts for assisting the members to say a few words about what has been most meaningful to them:

- "Even though we've been together only a short time, what are you learning about yourself in here?"
- "What are a few things that you think you're taking away with you from this session?"
- "Are you seeing any of your concerns reflected in others as they talk?"
- "What are you finding to be most helpful to you in here?" "And what is least helpful?"
- "Are there any ways in which anybody in this group can help you feel more secure in here?"
- "Was there anything that you didn't say earlier in this session that you'd like to briefly say before we quit?"
- "Are there any ways in which you'd like to be different in the next session than you were today?"

The main focus at the ending of the first few group sessions can be directed to a brief summary of what participants are experiencing as they are in the group. It is useful to shape the practice of getting members to reflect on what is occurring within the group. Even eliciting a few words from each person about the highlights of the session provides the pulling together that is so necessary as the group is taking shape. The point is to avoid ending abruptly with little or no closure.

Even during the initial sessions, members may get involved in work and feel as though they don't have enough time to finish what they started. If a client's work has been cut off either because the group ran out of time or because the client was distracted and lost momentum, the leader can help the member briefly state what he or she would have liked to accomplish from a piece of work. This sets the stage for returning to this work at a following meeting. Members need to learn that they will rarely "finish" with a problem they bring to the group, for there are always new facets of most issues to pursue. At the next session it is often possible to recapture the theme and the feeling even when the client believes that the opportunity has been lost. The leader can ask the client to start in again at the point where the interruption occurred, perhaps prompting with specific phrases. Without forcing the issue, leaders frequently find that the feelings return readily enough if the client will only begin speaking.

At the first few meetings, it is an important task for members to learn how to use the time they have allotted. Perhaps some of them will come to see that they wait too long before identifying a concern they'd like to pursue. Toward the end of a session the leader can teach a few brief ways of putting their personal agenda in clear terms and asking for time. Even during the initial stage, it is well for leaders to begin teaching members how to evaluate what they are giving and getting from their group. The last few minutes of a session can be devoted to some form of verbal or written assessment of that particular session. We now turn to ways in which members can best participate in this process of evaluation.

Techniques for Member Self-Evaluation

Early in the course of the group, the members need to learn how to assess their participation. The leader might ask: "How do you see yourself in this group at this time, and how do you feel about the way you are?" "If you continue being the same kind of member that you've been, how will you feel at the final session?" "In what ways, if any, do you see yourself as being different in this group than you are on the outside?" "What are some of the things that you like best about the way you've acted in this group?" "In what ways, if any, do you see yourself as having avoided working in this group so far, and what are you willing to do about this avoidance?" "What would you most like to change about the way you are or the way you feel in this group?"

These questions are excellent catalysts for focusing members on the direction in which they are moving. This technique invites members to change some of the ways in which they have either involved themselves in the group or stayed aloof. If participants say that they are dissatisfied with the way they have begun in the group, the leader can help them formulate specific strategies for changing.

What about those whose participation has been minimal? Understandably, most group leaders would like to have all the members of the group fully participate, and they sometimes force the issue. For example, some call on members and ask them what they think about the topic being discussed. Others ask each person in the group to answer a question. If leaders use these methods often, members may simply wait to be called on before they respond. If nothing seems to be happening, a far better technique is to address this issue directly in the group.

Leaders who are dissatisfied with the members' level of participation may also use structured techniques to keep things moving or to generate some activity. The use of these techniques can easily boomerang and contribute instead to the passivity of the participants, who begin to think that it is the leader's responsibility to keep things moving. The best technique here is to help members face those times when they are not involved and to challenge them to decide what they are willing to do for themselves.

A good technique for minimizing the possibility that group members will continue in nonproductive patterns is to have them evaluate their participation and progress in a group continually, perhaps by using a written form. It is a good practice to have members begin the process of self-evaluation during the first few group sessions. Then structure the group so that the participants can assess their functioning several more times. The following self-assessment form can be used for this evaluation. (An evaluation form designed for the end of a group is described in Chapter 7.)

• • • • • • • • • • • • • • • • • • •

Self-Assessment Form for Group Members

Rate yourself on the following statements using a scale from 1 to 5, with 1 being "almost never true of me" and 5 being "almost always true of me" as a group participant:

1. I am striving to be an active member in my group.
2. I am willing to become personally involved in this group and to share current issues in my life.
3. I see myself as willing to experiment with new behaviors in this group.
4. I make an effort to express my reactions pertaining to what is going on in my group.
5. I am able to talk about what may get in the way of my feeling safe in the group.
6. I am trying to let others know how they are affecting me at the time.
7. I strive to be clear about my goals and what I want from the group.
8. I listen attentively to others, and I respond to them directly.
9. I share my perceptions of others by giving them feedback on how I see them and how I am affected by them.
10. I am able to state my fears, reservations, and concerns about participation in the group.
11. I am willing to get involved in various exercises in the group.
12. I generally want to attend the group sessions.
13. I am able to provide support to others without coming to their rescue.
14. I take an active role in creating trust in the group.
15. I am open to considering feedback in a nondefensive way.
16. I seek to carry lessons learned in the group into my outside life.
17. I pay attention to my reactions to the group leaders and express what they are.
18. I avoid labeling myself and others in the group.
19. I avoid questioning others and giving them advice in the group.
20. I take responsibility for what I am getting from the group and what I am missing.

• • • • • • • • • • • • • • • • • • •

When we use a self-assessment device such as the one above, we discuss with the group the reactions of members to specific items on the form, paying particular attention to patterns and trends in the group.

Techniques for Leader Self-Evaluation

In addition to asking members to assess their progress in the group during the initial stage, leaders and co-leaders can evaluate their own effectiveness in the group at this time. The following form can be used at different times during the life of a group for self-assessment and also as a springboard for fruitful discussion between co-leaders.

• • • • • • • • • • • • • • • • • • • •

Self-Assessment Form for Leaders

Rate yourself on the following statements using a scale from 1 to 5, with 1 being "almost never true of me" and 5 being "almost always true of me" as a group leader:

1. I am generally enthusiastic about meeting my group.
2. I am willing to express my reactions to what is going on in the group.
3. I am able to help members clarify their goals and take steps to reach them.
4. I am able to understand members and to communicate this understanding to them.
5. I can challenge members in a direct way without increasing their defensiveness.
6. I am able to model desired behaviors in the group.
7. I am willing to take risks in pursuing hunches I have in working with members.
8. My timing of techniques is usually appropriate in that it does not interrupt the client's work.
9. I am sensitive to picking up clients' leads and following them rather than pushing members.
10. I am able to challenge my initial assumptions and perceptions regarding members.
11. My behavior in the group indicates that I have a basic respect for the members.
12. I am able to link the work of one member with that of another by picking up common themes.
13. I give thought to what I want to accomplish before I enter a session.
14. I allow adequate time for a summary and integration at the end of each session.
15. I am able to intervene effectively with members who engage in counterproductive behavior, without attacking them.
16. I provide support and positive reinforcement to members at appropriate times.
17. I usually work effectively with my co-leader, and when I don't, I am willing to admit it and talk about it at the appropriate time.
18. I make use of appropriate self-disclosure.

19. I use techniques with sensitivity to the client's cultural background.
20. I give thought to the techniques that I use in a group and have some rationale for using them.

•   •   •   •   •   •   •   •   •   •   •   •   •   •   •   •   •   •   •

Concluding Comments

During the initial stage of a group, the following are key tasks for leaders: to create an environment that helps build trust; to deal with members' fears, anxieties, and expectations; to be aware of their own persistent feelings and reactions; to encourage members to express persistent feelings and reactions regarding the group; and to help members go further in expressing personal reactions than they typically do. The early phase of a group is critical, because at this time the norms that will govern the group process are being shaped and the foundation of trust is being laid that will allow for productive work as the group moves forward. If the members' fears and reservations are not dealt with effectively as the group begins, the members are certain to encounter obstacles to developing genuine cohesion that will unite them. They will inevitably be stuck if they do not explore the fears that can keep them from fully participating.

Questions and Activities

1. How would you describe the characteristics of the initial stage of groups with which you are familiar? What techniques are you likely to use at the beginning of a group? What are your reasons for introducing these techniques?
2. Describe circumstances under which you think icebreaker techniques are in order. Describe techniques you might use to help members get acquainted, and give your reasons for introducing them. What potential disadvantages are there to using them?
3. Anxiety is typically present at the start of a group. Explain your rationale for being drawn to techniques that escalate this anxiety, dissipate it, or explore it. What considerations do you think are important in your response to anxiety?
4. Examine the room you are in right now. How might you best use this room for a group meeting? What are its liabilities, and how could you maximize its potential as a group setting? What objects in the room might serve as props for techniques? Try moving objects around, and try different seating arrangements. Discuss how these changes might affect the group.
5. How does the body posture of members influence others in a group?
6. We have said that structure is more appropriate at the initial stage of a group than later on. Do you agree?

7. Describe several techniques for use in the initial stage other than the ones we mention in this chapter. When do you think it might be appropriate to introduce these, and when might it be counterproductive?
8. What are some possible dangers or disadvantages in using exercises to create trust?
9. Under what circumstances, if any, would you engage in trust exercises? Explain.
10. Are you inclined during the early stage to urge members to make some declaration of what they want from the group? What advantages or disadvantages do you see to doing so, and what techniques do you think you might employ in this regard?
11. In the early stage of a group, do you favor using some structured exercises, or do you lean more to letting a group find its own way? Discuss.
12. You are asked to lead an involuntary group. Describe how you would deal with the issues you imagine would surface in the group, and discuss what techniques might be appropriate or inappropriate. How would you attempt to explain to the members the potential value of the group?
13. Enumerate several characteristics of resistance and the possible dynamics behind them, and create techniques that you think might be appropriate for working with them.
14. Would it be a goal of yours, ideally, to eliminate all resistance in a group? Is this possible? Explain your position.
15. How can you differentiate between a member's reluctance to trust that arises from cultural conditioning and resistance that stems from avoidance?
16. At the first meeting of a group, a member declares that you do not have the experience or ability to be leading. How might you deal with this challenge? Would you be inclined to introduce a technique at this point, and if so what might it be?
17. What techniques can you think of to get members focused at the beginning of each session?
18. How would you go about evaluating your own effectiveness as a leader? Describe some specific procedures.
19. What are some of the ways in which your modeling can lessen resistance among the members? What kind of modeling would you like to present in your dealing with resistant behaviors?
20. What balance would you like to provide between challenging members' fears and providing a supportive climate that will enable them to openly talk about their fears?

CHAPTER FIVE

Techniques for the Transition Stage

In this chapter we discuss some of the basic characteristics of a group during its transition stage, we focus on therapeutic ways of overcoming defensiveness and resistance, and we provide some techniques for dealing with difficult members.

Characteristics of the Transition Stage

Before a group can launch into extensive and productive work, typically it must go through a rather difficult transition phase. At this evolutionary period, members have the task of learning to recognize and deal with anxiety, resistance, and conflict. The members are:

- deciding whether they are willing to invest themselves fully in a group experience
- becoming aware of some feelings of which they were previously only dimly aware
- testing both the leader and other members to determine the safety level of the group
- observing the leader's behavior to determine the congruence between what the leader says and does
- feeling ambivalent about what they want from the group
- becoming more attuned to conflict that might be brewing within the group
- learning the importance of saying what they feel and think about the group

During this stage, it is the members' task to monitor their feelings and reactions and to learn to express them. It helps if members come to respect their resistances yet, at the same time, push themselves to challenge their tendencies toward avoidance. Members must learn how to confront others in a caring and constructive fashion and how to remain open and nondefensive in receiving feedback from others. If conflicts emerge, members will need to recognize them and develop the skills to work through them. Unrecognized conflicts will almost always lead to hidden agendas that result in a group's being stuck.

A central challenge for leaders at the transition stage is to develop interventions that help a group become a cohesive unit. Techniques need to be used with sensitivity and appropriate timing. One of the leader's tasks is to encourage members as they go through some difficult times. At the same time, leaders need to challenge members to face and resolve conflicts that evolve from the interactions in the room. Leaders demonstrate what they stand for by their actions. If they expect group participants to be honest, direct, and constructively confrontive, it behooves them to model these behaviors through their leadership.

Examples of Ways of Dealing with Defensive Behaviors

In this section we give a number of examples of typical avoidance behaviors—the defenses that members often employ in the transition stage of a group. For each of these behaviors we suggest approaches and techniques for dealing with it.

Having an external focus. Members in the transition stage of a group frequently focus on other people and on matters external to themselves. They may blame others either inside or outside the group for their inability to trust. For example, Darlene announces that she finds it difficult to be in the group because Charlie sits back and looks bored. Instead of looking at herself and her reactions, she focuses much of her attention on what he is doing, what he is not doing, and how she thinks he is "making" her feel. In this way she avoids dealing with her lack of involvement in the group. In this situation the leader might ask Darlene to speak directly to Charlie and tell him how she is affected by his presence in the group. Assume that she says "Charlie is so aggressive." The leader might ask: "What does his aggressiveness do to you? With what person in your life do you associate aggressiveness?" If Darlene is responding to Charlie as she does to someone close to her, perhaps she might reply: "Charlie, I'm scared of you, and I find myself reluctant to open up around you. You remind me of my ex-boyfriend." This technique of directing the focus toward clients who are making statements about others tends to encourage members to look at themselves and their part in the group.

Using impersonal and global language. John characteristically speaks in general terms and thus keeps himself shut off from other members. When, during one of the early sessions, the leader asks members to tell how they feel about being in the group, John says: "Nobody in here really wants to open up. Everyone is sitting back and waiting for the other guy to begin. People don't want to say what they think. They don't want to step on anyone's toes. Nothing is happening in here, because they're all putting up walls, and nobody wants to come out from behind these walls." Because John uses universal terms such as *nobody, they,* and *everyone,* others in the group have no idea whom he is talking about. Also, it's not clear whether he is including himself in this category, because he doesn't say that *he* has walls or that *he* is unwilling to open up.

Some possible tactics to help John become more personal and use more precise language are as follows:

- "John, I'd like you to say everything you've just said, but put 'I' in front of each of your sentences and see if there's a different feel to what you're saying."
- "Well, whom in here don't you want to open up to? What is it that you're thinking and not saying? What walls are you putting up, and against whom

- "I'm not clear about what you just said, John. Would you be willing to go around the group and say how you see each person in this group so far? It might help if you describe how you see each person as having walls, and tell each person how it feels to have these walls between you."
- "You keep talking about 'them.' Do you see yourself as one of 'them'? I have something I'd like to suggest as a way to begin to initiate some openness in this group. Please look at each of the other members, and imagine to yourself the walls that *you* might be building to keep your distance from each of us. [John does so. Then:] Pick one person in this room, and tell that person about any of the walls that are within you and what you imagine would happen if you took your wall down."
- "How about going around the circle and completing this sentence in a different way as you look at each person: 'One way I'd like you to be different in here so that I could be different is . . .'"
- "Tell us some of the ways in which the situation in this group seems like situations you find yourself in outside the group. How are you the same both in the group and in daily life?"
- "Could you replace each of the remarks you have made about other people's walls with a comment about some wall of your own?"

There are some other techniques for helping members narrow down their generalized statements. Below are a few generalizations we have heard in our groups, followed by interventions we are likely to make in an attempt to help the member become more concrete and focused:

- "Everyone is cautious about opening up." ("What are you cautious about in here?" "If you were to be less cautious right now, what might you say or do?")
- "Everyone in here is so hung up on talking about problems. Why can't people ever talk about the good stuff in their life instead of always focusing on the negative?" ("Who in particular talks about problems, and how does that person affect you?" "How would it be different for you if people did not dwell on problems?")
- "It seems that everyone who works in here always winds up crying or getting angry. Why is it that we're not believed unless we're in tears or unless we're frothing at the mouth?" ("What has it been like for you to be in a room where people show emotions?" "If you're adverse to displaying emotions as you work, how, specifically, would you prefer to be in this group?")
- "My problems are not as significant as other people's!" ("What problems of yours do you consider insignificant?" "What problems of others are more significant than yours?")

The art of skillful leadership involves confronting members in such a way that they will be more inclined to recognize defensive patterns such as focusing on others or consistently keeping themselves hidden by using impersonal and global language. If the confrontation is done by describing specific behaviors and not criticizing or labeling members, they are more likely to challenge their resistances. Participants such as John need help in seeing how they can be different.

Asking questions of others. A particular form of avoidance behavior that often manifests itself during the transition stage is asking questions of others. This defense drains away the energy from a group. Members using this defense demand that others make themselves known while they are keeping themselves safely hidden through their questions. For example, Jim perceives himself as an active and involved member merely because he bombards other members with questions. Even though the group is relatively young, he has already managed to ask personal questions of most of the members. He has asked others to give reasons for the feelings they have, and he has asked them whether they have tried this or that approach to solving a problem. His questions have usually interrupted group interaction.

Keeping in mind that Jim's style of questioning is a way of avoiding focusing on himself, the leader can use either of two techniques to get him to make personal references. The leader might ask Jim to go around the entire group and ask every question that he might possibly want to ask of everyone. (Members should not answer these questions.) The point of this exercise is to allow him to exaggerate his questioning behavior. When he's finished, the leader can ask him what the experience was like and can also ask him to tell each member what he might want from him or her. Alternatively, the leader can ask Jim to refrain from asking a question and instead to talk about what prompted him to ask the question. In this way, Jim can begin to disclose something of himself.

We do not mean to imply that all questions are manifestations of resistance. The types of questions that we would like members (and leaders) to refrain from asking are leading questions, questions that pry, or questions that are closed-ended and tend to cut off a member's exploration. We typically intervene when one member attempts to put thoughts into another person's head. For example, if a member says to a person who experienced child abuse "You must have hated your father," we might ask "How is hating your father an issue for *you*?" We would rather let members speak for themselves than have others suggest what a certain situation was like. We also try to abort questions that tend to go nowhere. When members ask questions, we typically invite them to at least briefly say why they are interested in hearing the answer.

Techniques for Dealing with Difficult Members

Members display certain difficult behaviors most conspicuously in the transition stage. The leader's early responses to them set a tone for the group. Members are observing the leader's behavior and are often silently deciding how much they can trust this person. In this section we discuss participants who are sometimes troublesome and give suggestions for dealing with them.

General principles.   The description of a member as "difficult" can be appropriate, or it can be the result of the leader's countertransference. Many leaders are sometimes unsure whether their reactions to an individual are valid or are rooted in their own idiosyncracies and unresolved conflicts. In general, we assume that our personal reactions to group members genuinely tell us something about the members. For example, if we find ourselves chronically annoyed with a certain behavioral pattern that Roberto displays, it may well be that he is repeating an old and familiar pattern that has been characteristic of his interactions with people since his early childhood. In fact, his behavior may be inviting people to shut him out or to dismiss him. These patterns are typically replayed in the interactions within the group, and we can learn a great deal about his dynamics by tuning in to our reactions to him. The perceptions we have of our clients are in many ways our best tools and the source of our techniques. For this reason, we allow ourselves, with some caution, to be guided by them. When others in the group share our reactions to an individual, their feedback can help us sharpen our awareness of a situation. Having said this, we want to add that countertransference reactions are often rooted in our own unfinished business. This means that we had better come to terms with our sources of vulnerability so that we do not get locked into a nontherapeutic alliance with a client whom we perceive as being problematic. Our willingness to explore our countertransference provides us with significant clues to the dynamics of both our clients and ourselves.

Because leaders have a responsibility to a whole group, they may decide to ask a difficult individual to stop coming. However, this solution can be damaging both to that individual and to the trust of the other members. The negative impact of the member on the group must be weighed against the impact of excluding him or her. Asking someone to leave the group should rarely be necessary, especially with adequate screening and preparation.

The greatest responsibility of a leader working with difficult members is to facilitate insight and growth, both for them and for the other members. To do so, the leader cannot rush in too quickly with ways of changing difficult members or "curing" them of their problematic behaviors. Initially, the leader should gather data, trying to ascertain whether the difficult members see themselves as causing problems for themselves or others, and what they might be attempting to communicate through their behavior. Both other members and the leader must be patient if resistance is to give way to more constructive behaviors. Those who exhibit problematic behaviors in the group can usually be dealt with in a direct and caring manner and can be given more of a chance to change in the group than they might be given in daily life. The basic purpose of a therapeutic group is to provide people with opportunities to see themselves in a new light and get a more accurate picture of how others perceive them. In the group context they can learn that they do not have to persist in a behavioral pattern that is leading them away from a path they would like to pursue. With the security afforded in a group, they can open themselves to taking risks and can dare to be different.

Leader modeling is extremely important here, for members do learn through this process. A common danger is to sum up quickly difficult members by attaching labels to them ("monopolizer," "group nurse," "seductive one"). Such labeling can encourage scapegoating, which only entrenches these members' styles by motivating them to retreat defensively into the identity given them. If resistant members are subjected to undue pressure or to uncaring attacks, the group can actually have a toxic effect, rather than a therapeutic one. A general guideline for leaders is to avoid saying "You are difficult" and to say instead "I am having difficulty with you." Leaders can then continue by pointing out specifically how and why they are being affected the way they are. For example, rather than saying "You're a storyteller, and by telling stories you're being a bore," the leader might say: "When you go on in such great detail about another person, I have a hard time paying attention to you. I'd much rather hear how you're affected by this person." Or the leader might put it more metaphorically: "I'd really like to be able to stay present with you and understand you, but it's not easy for me to get a sense of you when you describe things in so much detail. Even though I like walking in the forest, I'm getting lost in the woods."

When members know the specific behavior that the leader is having difficulty with, they can learn to observe this behavior in themselves. Then they are in a position to decide whether the behavior is a problem to them and also whether they are willing to change it. In the example given above, the member may realize that she typically loses others by going on in such a detailed fashion, yet she may decide that she doesn't want to change this aspect of herself. This is fine, but then she must be willing to accept the reality that her choice has consequences.

If leaders initiate feedback about a difficult member, they should do so in a manner that is sensitive, honest, and caring. They should realize that others in the group are likely to be observing their manner of confrontation, and thus it is well for them to be aware of what they are modeling for the members. Assume that most members see Doug as resistant and unapproachable and let him know this. The point is not to invite members to "dump on" Doug. Instead, they should be encouraged to provide him with their feedback and reactions but avoid ganging up on him. The leaders need to be careful to moderate the amount of feedback so that Doug does not get more than he can possibly assimilate at any one given time. If it appears that he is getting more than he can handle by way of feedback from others, the leader may intervene by saying "Perhaps Doug has had enough of our telling him who we think he is, and we can focus more on what is going on with each of us." Here, in order to offer an opening for further work, a leader might add "Before we do that, Doug, I'd like you to have an opportunity to respond to any of the feedback that you have received so far."

Although difficult members may experience any sort of feedback as criticism, it is nevertheless best for you, as the leader, to support the right of others to voice their reactions. However, you might also communicate strong supportive interest in and caring for the recipients of the feedback: acceptance of them, patience with them, and willingness to stay with them even though doing so is difficult. Your task as a leader is to help difficult members see and understand the difference between critical reactions and helpful reactions. You might let difficult members know that the feedback from others is compatible with the fact that these others care for them. If you honestly can do so, you might convey a willingness to accept difficult members as they are while at the same time offering them the opportunity for behaving in ways that would affect you differently. Thus, you can ask such members whether there is anything they would like to try doing differently or whether there is further work they would like to pursue.

We cannot give complete recipes for working with members who demonstrate difficult behaviors in a group. Your own reactions and inventiveness have to be the guide. We often say that it is important for both the leader and the members to talk about themselves when they are having difficulty with a member. Rather than focusing on judgments or interpretations of behavior that we perceive as being difficult, it is generally a good rule for us to talk about how we are affected in a personal way by these behaviors. In this regard, your ability to be honest, sensitive, caring, and timely is of the utmost importance. Often, it may be inappropriate to introduce any explicit technique at all beyond encouraging feedback and individual expression and offering interpretation of or comments on the group process.

In the transition stage, the group has not yet achieved the cohesion necessary to work through deeper problems. Thus, it may be inappropriate to promote much in-depth work with a difficult member who has received confrontive feedback. Even if this person is now ready to express some emotion or to work on some difficult and threatening material, the others in the group may not be ready for this work and may be excessively frightened by what they see as the consequences of giving feedback to one another. As we mentioned, the early interchanges with difficult members should be seen primarily as a source of valuable information for you to use later on. For example, you may want to ask difficult members whether the responses that they elicit from the group match the responses that they get in everyday life or that they got in childhood.

For the purposes of this book, we talk of "difficult members," but we don't address individuals in our groups in that way. From our vantage point, we do everything possible to avoid labeling people and to give them a chance to be different. We try to be patient even though their behaviors may strain our patience. We attempt to see various problematic behaviors as signs that people are struggling, and in this spirit we strive to understand what purpose their behavior is serving. The group setting provides an excellent format for people to see their own resistances in action. If they can avoid labeling themselves and putting themselves down in critical ways, they are more likely to feel the freedom to try out a different form of behavior. Techniques for working with a difficult member fall into two categories: those that focus on the member and those that focus on the responses of others to this member. Either focus can flow into the other, and you should be alert to this possibility. Techniques that focus on the difficult members include having them receive feedback in order to clarify the impact they have on others; having them exaggerate their behavior, perhaps to see it clearly, to tire of it, or to gain insight into its sources; having them try out a different behavior; and having them clarify that they are behaving as they want to behave. Techniques that focus on the responding members include asking them to comment to the difficult member on "other times I've felt as I feel with you now," on "times I feel outside the group as I feel with you now," or on "how I feel with you now and the options I have in dealing with these feelings."

During this kind of work, you need to be alert to the danger that group members will label difficult clients or that these clients will label themselves, particularly when they feel defensive, and then live up to these labels for the duration of the group. As we mentioned earlier, leaders need to be alert to the dangers of packaging people and reducing them to a simplistic label. If leaders steadfastly refuse to reduce people to some sort of stereotype, the members themselves are less likely to continue self-labeling. One of the purposes of a group is to provide a context in which participants can challenge self-defeating labels and begin to create positive identities. In this regard, techniques that invite difficult members to experiment with new forms of behavior are especially useful. In this way, members can not only think about ways in which they have embraced a limiting vision of themselves but also learn that they do not have to live by restrictive labels.

One way of stimulating difficult members to consider changing their behavior is to ask them whether they're getting from the group what they had hoped for when they signed up. If there is a discrepancy between the goals they have stated and how the leaders or the group members are seeing them, they can be invited to change their course. In this way leaders can check whether the difficult members themselves want to change. Are they interested in feedback? Do they think that they may be restricting themselves by accepting self-imposed labels or the labels others have given them? Do they want to take the risks involved in creating a different identity? If they decide that their current behavior is not working for them and they want to change it, the group is an excellent place for them to learn constructive behavior patterns.

Before suggesting specific techniques for dealing with difficult members in a group, we want to underscore some key points. Whom you experience as difficult depends on *you* as well as on your clients. You can trust your reactions while also acknowledging that these assessments reflect on yourself and on your own dynamics. You can seek to communicate your own responses to difficult members and can thus model this kind of feedback for other group members. You can also try to communicate a basic respect for the clients whose behaviors pose difficulties, even though the feedback given to them may be critical. Most important, you can be alert to how this kind of feedback may entrench clients in their problematic behaviors. You can communicate to these group members your openness to them as they are now and can encourage them to consider experimenting with ways of being different as a means of obtaining the goals they stated when they came to the group.

The person who is silent. Leaders need to model respect for silent members if they hope to create a climate that invites rather than forces members to participate. At the same time, it is important for leaders to communicate their interest in hearing from silent members and to be aware of the impact that quiet members may have on the others. In many groups other members will eventually comment on those who are silent. The quieter members may appreciate the interest that others take in them, if leaders wait for the group to initiate this feedback rather than give it themselves. If leaders do initiate the topic of silence, they can express their hope that those who have not participated are getting what they want from the group. They can then encourage silent members to discuss what is inhibiting them. They can also inform quiet members of the impact they have on others, particularly when others seem to be inhibited for fear of being judged by those who do not participate. Finally, leaders can express an interest in whether the silence of these members within the group is indicative of their style outside the group, and they can remind silent members of their opportunity to try out a different way of being.

Both group leaders and the other participants can make the mistake of pushing the silent client to open up without discovering why the person is being silent, and they can make the mistake of focusing on the quiet member and using many means of drawing this individual out. As a result, the silent member often becomes increasingly quiet, withdrawn, and resistive. In many cases, silence is not a defense but a learned behavior that is congruent with the client's cultural background. For instance, Quan says very little in her group, and in spite of the repeated attempts of other members and the leader to get her to say more, she remains a polite listener. Eventually the group discovers that in Quan's culture it is considered rude to talk about oneself; doing so would be seen as being self-centered. Thus, when she asks questions of others, she is doing what works for her in her family and larger culture. After a while, she lets the group know that she does not judge others for talking in very personal ways about their families but that for her to do so would be most difficult. She has been taught that it is shameful to expose the family's "dirty linen" in public. Quan does tell the group that she does not like being seen as "the quiet one" in so many social circles. She sometimes envies people who can be free and outgoing, and she would like to become a bit more outspoken—but it is difficult.

A technique for exploring the reactions of active participants to one who is silent is to encourage them to tell one another or the silent member (depending on how threatening the leader judges this to be) how they feel about having expressed themselves openly around someone who has not reciprocated. Exercises of this type can be introduced in a way that minimizes embarrassment to those who are typically silent. Or the feedback to the silent members can be confrontive to challenge them to share more of themselves. We cannot give a blueprint for what is appropriate here. You may want to be more confrontive with someone whose silence is manifestly hostile and disruptive and more supportive with someone who is a part of the group but is shy or inhibited.

A technique for working with several silent members is to ask them to form an inner circle and then to say as much as they are willing to about their being silent. They can be asked to talk about what it has been like for them to be in the group so far. The chances are that they have been very observant and that they can share openly what they have been thinking and feeling. The leader should make sure that these people are interested in doing the exercise.

A variation of the preceding technique focuses on the active members. They can form an inner circle and talk about their feelings about being left out of what the members who are silent are thinking. This exercise gives those in the inner circle an opportunity to discuss how it is for them to disclose in the presence of those who do not. It also gives those who are verbally inactive (in the outer circle) feedback about the impact of their silence on others.

As a further illustration of possible techniques for dealing with the member who is habitually silent, we now describe Donna's behavior and apply some of the principles we've just been discussing. When the leader asks her how she has experienced the group so far, she shrugs her shoulders and says: "It's hard for me to talk in a group. I prefer being a listener. I don't like feeling forced to talk and to say what I think. I learn a lot just by listening to what others in here are saying." One approach is to ask Donna whether she'd like to be different from the way she is. Would she like to be more verbal in the group? Is her listening style satisfactory to her? Is she getting what she wants by being silent in the group?

Or the leader can say: "Donna, I'd guess you don't realize how powerful an impact your silence has on me. For example, I find myself fantasizing that you don't approve of how I'm leading this group, and I wonder whether other members might tell you some of their fantasies about how you see them?"

Or the leader can ask Donna to talk about what it is like for her to be in the group. How does it feel for her to be a listener? How is her behavior characteristic of the way she is outside the group? What factors is she aware of that keep her from saying what she is thinking and feeling in the group? By answering these questions, Donna is letting people know something about her.

Donna may eventually say that she talks little in the group because she doesn't know what is expected of her, that she has never been in a group before, and that she'd like to say more but finds herself being inhibited and doesn't want to call attention to herself. She may say that the others seem to know what they want from the group but that she still doesn't know what to work on. One technique to use here is to ask Donna to look at each person in the group and complete the sentence "When I look at you, I think that you expect me to . . ." She may add, for example, ". . . talk as much as you do," ". . . come up with some problem to work on in this group," ". . . become involved in this group or decide to leave," ". . . tell you that I'm not judging you and that I accept what you're saying," ". . . show some feelings," or ". . . tell you something about myself." Donna's statements provide rich material for the leader to tap into. After she has made the rounds and dealt with her projections, she can be asked what this experience was like and what she learned from the exercise. Then members may want to spontaneously offer her feedback about their expectations of her. It is important not to short-circuit the process of Donna's struggle. If she were to say "I wonder what people think of me, and I wonder if I'm living up to what others expect of me," we would generally not facilitate by encouraging members to share their reactions too quickly. We prefer her to work with her own projections and her own internal dynamics before she seeks reassurance from others.

Another technique for working with expectations is to focus on Donna's expectations of others. She can go around the group and complete the sentence "Looking at you now, I expect you to . . ." These two exercises can be combined by asking her first to go around the group saying what each person expects of her and then to go around making statements about what she expects of each person.

If Donna lets us know that her silence is something that troubles her and that she would like to change it, we can ask her to talk more about how it has been for her to be in this group up to now, having said little. We can invite her to pursue any of these questions: "What are some things you're thinking and telling yourself when you want to participate but don't?" "How do you imagine this group might be different for you if you were to say more?" "You say you've been silently observing and learning. Would you tell us what you've been learning? Perhaps you could address specific people in here, letting each of them know what you're learning from them." Any of these questions could facilitate Donna's work in understanding the ways in which she inhibits herself. She can begin to see the functions her silence serves.

A final suggestion for working with a silent member like Donna is to ask her to close her eyes and imagine that the way she has begun the group—namely, assuming the role of listener—is the way she will continue until the end of the group. She can be directed to imagine that this is the last session. What is she thinking now? What has she gotten from the group? How does she feel about her level of participation? What might she be saying to herself? This technique is designed to get her to think about the pattern of behavior she is developing in the group and to project this pattern into the future.

It gives her a chance to examine how she may be allowing expectations that she imagines others to have of her to interfere with her participation in the group, and it gives her a chance to declare what she is willing to do differently if she doesn't like what she sees when she closes her eyes.

The person who monopolizes.   While the member who is silent is likely to be challenged by the group, the person who monopolizes group time is often less likely to be effectively confronted. Some leaders prefer to let group members struggle with a monopolizer in their own way. If you prefer having a group in which many take an active role, however, you may choose to intervene. Here again a technique may not be called for; simply sharing your observations and reactions may suffice. Techniques that draw out the reactions of others are appropriate here, because those who monopolize are already getting plenty of time. You should guide this feedback to guard against inhibiting the talkative individuals too much. You can say that those who speak a lot are valued for what they are contributing and that you hope they will continue to be active while others speak up as well. A powerful technique to use with clients who monopolize, as well as with other difficult members, is to videotape or tape-record their work. By providing direct feedback, the tapes allow these members to evaluate how they present themselves. In addition, highly structured techniques such as using a stopwatch or an egg timer may be appropriate.

Another technique that may be useful with monopolizing individuals and with other difficult members is to recommend that they persist in their behavior. Thus, by saying "I'd be interested in seeing what would happen if you talked *more* often," you can often challenge these members to talk less. You can then comment on this response and explore it. But this approach would need to be gauged against the potential outcomes for a particular member and the trust level of the group.

A difficult client is often able to assimilate feedback that is given caringly but humorously. A leader can, for example, urge other members to give imitations of how a monopolizer appears to them. However, a word of caution is in order here. If sufficient trust has not been established, there is likely to be a boomerang effect. The person who is getting the feedback may feel put down and exhibit another equally problematic behavior or may increase his or her monopolizing behavior.

The person who is sarcastic.   Clients are not challenged to deal with their feelings as long as they continue to express them indirectly. Voicing anger directly is constructive, but expressing anger in a disguised form through sarcasm is not. Jan says "I'm not as high-class as Marie, but I dress nicely." Jan is probably saying indirectly that Marie is snooty, but she isn't facing her hostility toward Marie, and Marie feels vaguely affronted by Jan without knowing exactly what she has been told. If this sarcasm is a persistent trait of Jan's, it can poison the trust and sharing of the group. In addition to eliciting feedback and responses from other group members, such as asking Marie what she thinks Jan has just told her, you might introduce techniques to teach Jan directly how she can express straightforwardly the anger she evidently feels. A different approach is to ask her to make a sarcastic remark to every member of the group and then to comment on how it was sarcastic and what it indirectly revealed about herself. If she is ready for in-depth work, you can introduce a technique that explores how and from whom she learned her sarcastic style and why she needs to disguise her anger.

The person who habitually focuses on others. Members who do not give of themselves and who avoid talking in personal terms often cause difficulty in a group. This category includes self-appointed group leaders, those who seek to bandage the pain of others without allowing them to explore it, those who constantly offer advice, those who question others endlessly, those who assert that they no longer have the problems others are struggling with, and those who bestow the pearls of wisdom they have gleaned from their experience. All these members tend to give the impression that they have no struggles of their own, thus providing a less-than-supportive environment for those who are trying to be open about their problems.

Like the silent members, these clients are likely to be challenged by others in the group. It is a good idea for the leader to encourage other members who are feeling inhibited to express and work with their reactions. This feedback in itself is often all that is needed to cause the difficult members to focus on themselves. In addition, leaders can teach group members that, paradoxically, we sometimes give more to others when we let them profit from the time we take for ourselves than when we direct our attention to trying to help them directly.

These techniques are not intended to take away from members a sense of altruism or a desire to help others but to show them that the group is seeing only one side of them: their need to give advice, to give comfort, or to take care of others. The goal is for such members to come to see the group as a place where they can get something for themselves, where they can learn to receive from others, and where they can decide whether their giving style is working for them or whether they might not profit from adding other dimensions to themselves.

One technique for encouraging change is to ask the member being described to go around and give each person one piece of advice and then to say "And from you I want . . ." This technique allows the client to do what comes easily, which is to give advice. It also asks the client to do something difficult, which is to ask for something from each person. Of course, this technique works only when the member wants to at least consider changing the type of behavior being described.

Techniques for Dealing with Conflict

A transition stage characterized by conflict and the expression of a variety of negative reactions is typical in the development of a group. When a group is in transition, creating and maintaining trust continues to be a major task.

As resistances are manifested, it is essential to understand the purpose and function that these behaviors serve. During the transition stage, members often challenge one another and are challenged by the leader. As a part of the group's striving toward its own independence, leaders are also frequently challenged, as you will see later in this chapter.

Conflict is related to the issue of difficult members because many conflicts result from the failure to deal directly with these clients. Also, the presence of difficult members in a group often escalates conflict. If a group is to progress, this conflict must be recognized and dealt with openly.

Intermember conflicts. The following typical comments characterize the transition stage:

- "I feel that Fred is intimidating."
- "I don't like all this hostility."
- "Why do we focus so much on the negative?"
- "Some people are monopolizing the group time."
- "There's a lot of intellectualizing going on."
- "I don't belong here, because my problems are not as severe as those of everyone else."
- "I'm bored."
- "We're not talking about real issues."
- "Some people sound as if they have it all together."
- "I have a hard time opening up around Lawrence, because he reminds me of my boyfriend."
- "George is slouching and looks bored."

These remarks are, for the most part, indirect, focused away from the speaker, and negative. Your response to virtually all these statements might be designed to change indirect confrontation to direct confrontation. Encourage the speaker to replace "some people," "he," and "she" with a personal focus on themselves. Suggest that Sally tell Lawrence about herself and how she responds to him rather than telling him how he is or who he is.

The group must experience and work through this stage rather than retreating to insincere politeness, but how conflicts at this stage are handled is extremely important. A group often finds a scapegoat and directs excessive and unconstructive negative feedback to that individual. One technique here is for leaders to direct attention away from the scapegoat by giving feedback to the group as a whole, describing the nature and stage of the group process as they see it and commenting on the importance of struggling with the emerging conflict in an honest way. Here are some other techniques for dealing with conflict:

- "If you're bored, what is not happening for you?"
- "Please tell us what you were thinking and feeling before you said you felt bored."
- "Please sit directly in front of Lawrence. Tell him how you feel in his presence. [Sally does so. Then:] Now would you be willing to tell Lawrence

about experiences you have had with people in your life that your experience with him reminds you of?"
- "Would you pretend for a moment that you're George? Slouch the way
he does, and talk about your fantasy of what he is feeling and thinking,
as if you were in his place."
- "Would you like to say, Fred, how it feels to be told you are intimidating?"
- "You claim you don't belong in the group, Ann, because your problems
are less severe than those of the others. Please tell each member of the
group how you differ from him or her. Afterward, I'll invite them to express their feelings about what you've said."
- "Sally, you said your father was very critical. Would you assume his role
and continue with your criticisms of Lawrence?"

In the last example the leader's response is fairly interpretive and is inappropriate unless the surrounding context is right. Furthermore, this intervention tends to take the focus away from the conflict in the room. It could be
appropriate at this stage, however, because it could lead members to explore
their individual dynamics when expressing their reactions to others. Also,
it is clearly fitting to ask a client to elaborate on associations if the client has
already indicated that this connection exists ("Lawrence reminds me of my
boyfriend").

In general, leaders should check out the reactions of the client receiving
the criticism but work primarily with the person giving it, partly to teach
members that they are in a group chiefly to explore and express themselves
rather than to change others. What a leader models at this point can stimulate
the group's progress. A leader can demonstrate the difference between "telling Lawrence who you think he is" and "telling Lawrence how you feel in
response to him." We prefer that members talk about how they are affected
by Lawrence rather than telling him how he is.

In addition, the leader can give Lawrence an opportunity to say how
he feels about what he has been told. If he seems resistant to this feedback,
the leader can emphasize that she hopes he will consider what was said but
that he need not accept it. She should be alert to the group's haranguing
him or trying to force their feedback on him and could comment that the
group members have found a scapegoat instead of keeping the focus on
themselves. If, however, Lawrence gives his permission for further work and
is interested in exploring the validity of the feedback, the leader could encourage him to talk about how it is to be the sort of person others have suggested he is. For example, if he has been told that others experience him
as judgmental and he agrees that others often see him this way or that, indeed, he is this way, the leader can ask him to exaggerate this characteristic
by talking to the group in a judgmental manner.

Ann, who said she didn't belong in the group because her problems
weren't as severe as everyone else's, did focus on herself, but her remarks
often turn out to be a disguised way of talking about others: "I don't belong
here, but you folks do; you are all sick." Here you might first encourage her
to go ahead and talk about the others—that is what is going on anyway—and

then bring the focus back, more honestly, to her. For example, she may be terribly afraid of having problems like those of others in the group. Once this feeling becomes evident, you could explore this fear and related fears concerning what might happen if she allowed herself to look at conflicts in her life that she habitually glosses over.

Techniques for Exploring Common Fears and Resistance

We often pick up on a sentence or a phrase that members utter, and we develop a technique that can help them pursue more fully a fear that could easily stop them from interacting in the group. For instance, in the first scenario to follow, a member prevents herself from doing productive work because she allows herself to be stopped by her fear that some people in the group might not approve of and like her. Our task is to help a member such as Laura see how she is stopping herself and provide her with a gentle impetus to get beyond her resistance.

"I'm afraid you won't like me." Group members are likely to feel that they will not be liked if they are open with their thoughts and feelings. Laura is a member of an open group. During the fourth meeting, some of the members tell her that although she has participated, they do not think she has shared much of herself. She replies that she's afraid that if she says more, she won't be liked. Another member, Ruth, observes that at times Laura seems to be looking on disapprovingly when other members reveal something about themselves, and as a result she feels that Laura may not like the rest of the group. Laura says that she does indeed find herself thinking critically about other people.

Here the leader can ask Laura to voice some of her reactions to each of the members of the group and encourage her to include critical comments. In every instance Laura's remarks may be critical of the person to whom they are directed, but she may also display much insight and genuine caring. She can thus discover that her criticalness is appreciated and is constructive without being devastating. This outcome often occurs when people such as Laura voice the critical thoughts they are so frightened of. Ruth's feedback to Laura is helpful, but the leader may be struck by the fact that Ruth also seems to convey an attitude of disapproval. This is a good opportunity to pursue work with both clients at once.

There is another way to work with Laura's fear that she will not be liked. You could ask her: "Who in this room do you think won't like you? What is going on in here that makes you think you won't be liked?" The rationale for this approach is that she may sense that someone doesn't like her. She could be having a transference reaction to a particular person, and it could be facilitative to ask her "Who do you imagine will not like you?" In working with Laura it would probably be best to focus first on who wouldn't like her and what this person might not like about her. This could produce some fertile material for group interaction.

"There's someone here I don't like." In a workshop we conducted, a participant, Bernie, announced that there was one person with whom he did not want to be in a subgroup. We made a tactical error by not doing more with Bernie's remark and paid for it later, because the group was especially slow to develop trust and cohesion. Since he did not say specifically whom he disliked, everyone else was left to wonder. We were not willing to confront him directly at the time, because we sensed that this particular group might perceive us as too directive and threatening if we insisted that he specify whom he disliked.

One approach a leader might take is to say something like: "Bernie, I'm sure what you just said has had an effect on people in this room, and I hope you won't stop there. You've made a good start, so say more. What is it about this person that you're having a reaction to? How does this person affect you? With all these reactions you have, you will get in your own way if you don't say more." The leader recognizes that what Bernie is not saying will certainly inhibit both his own participation and the participation of others in the group. The leader's techniques are designed to challenge him to take the risk involved in being specific. If he does this, members can deal with him directly, and there is an opportunity to resolve potential conflicts.

"I'm afraid to look at what I'm really like inside." As a symbolic way of exploring Julie's fear of inner conflict, we might begin by saying to her: "I'd like for you to stand by that closet door over there and pretend that some hidden dimensions of yourself are inside. Maybe you could open the door just a crack, peek inside, and report to the group as you do so about what you suspect may be inside." Or: "Maybe you could stand inside the closet. As you peer out at the rest of us, talk about some of what you fear may be in there that you are reluctant to let come out."

There's no telling in advance where this exercise might go. People can be insightful when in a playful mood, and Julie may quickly identify in a half-joking manner some of the fears she has about what might be locked up inside her. Or she or others in the group may have had a childhood experience with closets—being put in one as a punishment for having expressed feelings unacceptable to their parents, for example; such experiences can lend power to this exercise. In either case, by urging Julie to physically move in the room to undertake this suggested activity, we make her a tangible focus of group work and feedback, a real part of the group.

Other techniques could be used here. We might ask Julie to list all the fears she can spontaneously come up with. She could make the list by completing these sentences: "One thing I'm afraid of is . . . And this reminds me of another thing I'm afraid of, which is . . ." In this form of free association we are encouraging Julie to identify the specific objects of her fears.

"I can't see why we have to share our feelings." James makes this remark after there has been much intensity in the group. The leader can begin by finding out whether anyone else in the group has the same doubts. Those who do can sit in the center of the room and talk to one another about why it is useless to express so much emotion. This technique gives these people an opportunity to express some of the resistance they are experiencing, which might otherwise inhibit the group's progress. This technique also gives these people, indirectly, an opportunity to do the very thing they are concerned about: express some of what they are feeling. The leader can ask them afterward how they feel about having expressed these concerns and can thus encourage them to go even further. Another way to pursue this exercise is to ask these members to talk about what they have experienced or have been taught about expressing feelings. Another technique is to set up a dialogue between members who are reticent and those who have shown some emotional intensity. After a few minutes, these people can exchange sides and try to put themselves in each others' place.

When a member like James voices a concern about expressing feelings, you should be aware of several possible dynamics. James's own way of recognizing his feelings may work well for him and yet be less dramatic than the way others in the group recognize their feelings. It may be that he is expressing widespread group resistance. If so, this resistance needs to be explored. Or he may be afraid of his own feelings. In this case you might use one of the following techniques:

- "When in your life might you have learned that it is better to keep feelings to yourself?"
- "What feelings do you find to be particularly troublesome?"
- "Whose voice do you hear inside your head when you do express your feelings? What do you tell yourself at these times?"
- "If your parents were here, what would they say about all this expression of emotion?"
- "Would you be willing to tell each of the people here whom you have experienced as fairly emotional what you get from keeping to yourself the sorts of feelings they have expressed?"
- "Go around to each person, and speculate on what he or she would think of you if you expressed more emotion."
- "Would you talk about the worst things you could imagine happening if this group were to continue expressing so much feeling?"
- "Suppose you decided today to keep your feelings and physical symptoms very much to yourself. How do you picture your life ten years from now if you stick to this decision?"

You may or may not want to go looking for relevant childhood lessons at this point, but when a client is fearful of the affect expressed in a group, usually you can be sure that these lessons are relevant. Many people were taught as children to inhibit their emotions, and others witnessed devastating consequences of the expression of feeling. They may have accepted parental injunctions that they should "stuff" their feelings or that they should keep "a stiff upper lip." As children, if they dared to release any emotions, they may have met with stern reactions from their parents. In addition to what they learned from their family, they may be hearing cultural injunctions against feeling. Consequently, they may have decided to stifle all of their emotions lest they meet with disapproval from others. Any of the above exercises is likely to bring to the surface the early decisions that James may have reached about the dangers of letting feelings be known.

"We seem stuck in our group." When members make such a statement, leaders, in addition to looking at their own responsibility, need to explore the dynamics in the group itself that are slowing it down. If techniques are used at all at a point like this, the objective should be to address the reasons for the impasse and not to get things moving artificially. Our aim would be to encourage members to verbalize what they are thinking, perhaps with an exercise such as the following: "Maybe each of you could say a bit about whether we *do* seem stuck and, if so, how this has happened." Creative use of the metaphors that members voice may be helpful. For instance, utilizing the phrasing of Joanna, who says "We seem to be stuck in the mud," the leader might propose: "How would it be if each of us commented on where we're stuck in the mud? What's bogging us down here?"

But with or without the help of an explicit technique, the crucial thing is to address what is going on. A lot is happening in the group, but the problem is that members are not expressing what they are thinking and feeling; on some level they are choosing to remain stuck. Employing any technique to reduce the anxiety in the room takes the responsibility away from the members to go beyond the point of being stuck. A better technique is simply to challenge the members to say out loud some of the things they've been saying to themselves. This tactic should bring into the open key issues that have been hidden and should provide an opportunity for a discussion and resolution of some of these issues. Although many members may not have voiced their concerns up to this point, the leader may now hear statements such as those given below from the members.

Sharon says: "I'm still not willing to say too much in here, because every time I do, people seem to jump on me. So I've decided to sit back and watch the game." The leader can begin by exploring with Sharon how she sees the group as a game. She can be asked to talk about what she has been watching as well as to describe her personal reactions. She can be asked to be specific by saying whom she perceives as "jumping on" her. This approach might provide an opportunity for the leader to discuss with the group the difference between attacking and caring confrontation. Perhaps Sharon is defensive about even constructive confrontation. Or perhaps the leader or some of the members are being overly aggressive. This technique allows the leader to discover whether the block is within Sharon or whether this is a block for most members. If confrontation is generally being handled poorly by the group, the leader needs to both model and teach a more effective way of confronting.

Janice says: "I'm afraid to really let myself get involved in this group, because I don't want to cry. If I begin to cry, I just might open up so much hurt that I won't be able to close up the wounds. So I'm keeping myself reserved." Here, if Janice is willing to take the risk, she can talk about her most terrible fantasy of what would happen if she were to cry. What might it be like for her to open up wounds that she thought were healed? By pursuing this fantasy, Janice can get a clear idea of whether she wants to continue holding herself back.

Grant announces: "For me this group is scary. I'm afraid to open up for fear that if I do, I just might go crazy." The leader can invite Grant to explore what he imagines it would be like for him if he were to go crazy in the group. He might be afraid of becoming angry, of hurting someone, of being perceived as different, or of losing control. These more specific fears can then be worked with. Or Grant can explore his original fear in depth by disclosing to the group what he imagines it would be like for him to actually go crazy. What would he be feeling? What would others think of him? How would he deal with what he had opened up in the group when he left the session? Again, these leads are all good ones for the leader to follow up, assuming Grant is willing to do so.

Dorothy declares: "I don't seem to know what I want from this group. I have a hard time really deciding what to talk about when I come here. Things seem to be going pretty well in my life, and right now I'm not aware of any pressing problems I need to bring up." She may be stuck because she no longer wants to continue with the group. She may not feel a need to explore problems, or she may not yet be able to identify specific areas of her life that she'd like to change. Both of these issues can be fruitfully pursued in the group, and as a result she may make the decision to withdraw.

Don says: "Frankly, I feel we're not getting anywhere as a group because we never stick with a person long enough to solve that person's problem. What good does it do to just talk? If we're not providing solutions for problems we bring up, what good is the group?" In this case, the leader can deal with Don's expectation that a group is a place to solve problems; he may be expecting simple solutions to complex problems. The leader needs to assert that a group's purpose is not to solve problems but to give members a chance to identify personal issues and to explore various facets of these issues. Too narrow a focus on problem solving can encourage members to give advice and patch people up, which has the effect of discouraging them from expressing feelings.

Molly says: "So what should I do about my problem? I just don't know whether I should file for divorce or settle for the way things are in my marriage. I don't seem able to make this decision for myself, and I'm looking to the group to give me advice." Molly may be feeling stuck because she doesn't see herself any closer to a decision than when she entered the group. Here is a good opportunity to work with her expectations of members and leader. She may be hoping for an answer outside herself because she is unwilling to commit herself to a decision and accept its consequences or because she does not trust herself enough to make decisions. One way of getting her through her impasse is to have her look at the degree to which she is willing to take personal responsibility for her life. She may be using the group to justify whatever action she does take, or she may be asking the group to make the decision for her so that she will not be accountable. These issues must be explored before Molly can hope to resolve her dilemma.

These examples illustrate that indeed a lot is going on within the group. Members are stuck largely because of their unwillingness to disclose to the group some of the things they are experiencing and telling themselves. Whenever a member speaks for the entire group, we would inevitably challenge this person by asking: "How are *you* stuck? How does this apply to *you*?" Our interventions are geared to getting the member who makes a global declaration about the group's being stuck to take responsibility for his or her own feelings by personalizing the statement. The basic technique here consists of encouraging people to bring out into the open their thoughts and feelings about how they are experiencing the group. This technique provides plenty of material to work with, and the group no longer stays on a plateau.

"I don't feel safe in here." Jill declares to the group that she sees others as able to openly share what they feel and talk about themselves in ways that are not easy for her. She adds that she'd like to be able to let others know what she's like, but somehow she just doesn't feel safe doing so. She agrees to work on what is blocking her.

The leader can use a number of techniques to help Jill explore ways in which the group could become a safer place for her. One direct approach is to simply say: "Jill, I wonder whether you can tell us what it's been like in here for you? Would you be willing to tell us what you've been feeling about the climate? How has it been for you to feel that you've had to hold yourself back?" These questions give Jill an opportunity to disclose what she has been feeling as a member of the group, without putting her on the spot to talk about other personal issues.

If Jill is willing to say what she has been experiencing as a member of the group, this will probably provide many leads for further work. She may acknowledge her fear of being judged by some of the members. When asked to select one of the members, she picks Peter. The leader can then say: "Jill, would you be willing to look at Peter and tell him all the things that you imagine he'd be saying to himself or to others if you were to let him know who you are? It would help if you could say everything that you can think of without rehearsing. Just list all the judgments you can imagine Peter making of you." This technique can provide the basis for a dialogue between Peter and Jill. The rationale is to give her an opportunity to say what she is silently ruminating about and to allow her to check out her assumptions. Jill may be thinking that Peter is highly critical of her, that he doesn't like her, and that he could not possibly be interested in her. His actual thoughts, however, may be that he'd like to hear more from her and that he misses her participation in the group. Unless she checks out her assumption, she will continue to operate as though it were true.

After the leader has worked with Jill, he might ask others in the group whether they feel the way she does. If one or more members do feel unsafe in the group, they, along with Jill, can form an inner circle and tell one another all the ways in which they perceive danger in the group and how it feels for them to be in the group. They can also talk about what they could do to make the group a safer place for them. Other members can then provide feedback and reactions based on what they heard from the inner circle.

An alternative strategy is for the leader to ask Jill to zero in on what appears to be an underlying irrational belief—that everyone is judging her and that she must gain everyone's approval—and to evaluate the validity of this belief. The leader can suggest that she give the group a lecture on the supreme importance of being alert to the judgments of others and on ways to gain universal approval. The leader can encourage her to say how horrible it would be if everyone were not to win this approval. After her lecture, the leader can ask her to explore questions such as these:

- "Who told you that it is absolutely essential that everyone approve of you? Does this assumption prevent you from being the person that you want to be?"
- "What price are you paying to gain the universal approval that you are seeking? Is it worth it?"
- "Is what others think of you more valid and important than what you think of yourself?"
- "How much sense does it make to hold beliefs about others that you do not check out?"

Another approach is to ask Jill to monitor her behavior during the week and to make notes of the times and situations in which she feels judged. She can also record what she does in such situations, what she feels, and what she tells herself. By making such notes, she may become aware of how her inner dialogue is creating her feeling of being judged. She can bring her notes to the group and report on the patterns of her behavior that became apparent to her. She can also think about how she might behave differently in these situations and then set up role-playing situations in the session to practice specific alternative behaviors.

For example, Jill reports that she experienced much anxiety when she took her car back to a shop that had charged her $150 for a poorly done tune-up. Although she was barely able to make it back to the mechanic with her sputtering engine, she quickly became apologetic and did not insist that he fix the car without further charges. Consequently, it cost her an additional $50, which she felt was unjustified. All the way home she told herself how quickly she had backed down and how her desire to gain the mechanic's approval had kept her from being as direct as she would have liked to be. In the group session, Jill can practice assertive behavior with the mechanic through role playing. Others can give her clear feedback on specific aspects of her behavior that contribute to her ineffective style in getting what she wants when she thinks she is right. The members can coach her in saying certain phrases, using a different posture, or changing the tone of her voice. Along with this assertiveness training in the group, she can also be asked to evaluate her underlying beliefs and thoughts to determine how they keep her from being the direct person she says she would like to be.

This example and the preceding one indicate that the issue of trust is not settled during the initial stage of the group. It may surface again and again in the group's history, often following periods of intense emotion. The usual signals are silence, lifelessness, or superficiality. Leaders should remain alert to clues that trust is, once again, an unexpressed concern within the group and seek means for giving it expression in order to move on to personal issues. Jill, for example, first had to deal with her lack of trust— both in herself to express what she was thinking and feeling and in others in the group—before she could openly discuss personal matters. By working on trust, she freed herself to report "failures" without being frozen by the fear that others would think badly of her.

"I can't identify with anyone here."   Sam, a retired executive, came to the group because of pressure from his wife, who complained of his being unfeeling. He rarely makes contributions in the group except to say what he thinks is wrong with others and how they ought to pull themselves together and be done with their problems. He usually looks critical and impatient. Finally, Patricia says she wishes that he would open up more. He replies: "I can't really identify with anyone in here. Maybe it's the age difference between me and most of you, or maybe it's just that you people have different sorts of concerns from mine." Here, the leader can suggest exercises such as these:

- "Tell everyone in this group, Sam, how you're different from him or her, and then add 'and I'm very different from you.' "
- "Walk outside the group to intensify your sense of distance. Then talk to us about how you feel being outside."
- "Stand on a chair, above everyone, and tell us how you are different from each of us."
- "Pick the person you feel the most like, and tell that person how the two of you are alike."
- "Now pick the member you identify with least, and tell that person how you are not alike."
- "Imagine that you're driving home alone after this group meeting. Talk out loud as you reflect on how different you are from everyone in this group."
- "Again, let yourself imagine that you're driving home tonight. Assume that in some ways you are really very much like everyone in here. Find one way in which you could identify, even in a small way, with each person. Talk out loud as you get this picture in focus."

These techniques encourage Sam to check out his assumptions. His lack of identification with others may be a defense. He may reveal the loneliness that results from being unable to identify with anyone, or he may get some insight into what he gains from being an outsider.

After completing a go-around, the leader, Peggy, can ask Sam whether he feels any different and whether he is interested in exploring separateness from others as a possible theme in his life. He tells Peggy that he does feel lonely in his marriage. She might then say: "Could you pick out the person here who most reminds you of your wife, and talk to her about what you have been saying to us? Perhaps you could say to her some things you haven't said before." Sam may say: "I can't do that. No one here reminds me of my wife. I don't see what good this would do."

In dealing with Sam's resistance, Peggy should be aware of how Sam is affecting her and should ask herself how much investment she has in leading him further than he seems to want to go. She may need to remind herself that Sam has spent a lifetime not expressing himself. Here again, a good technique is to join him in the resistance: "OK, Sam. No one here is going to make you do anything you don't want to do. You are going to have to tell me what you want." Or if Peggy has a hunch that he wants some prodding, she can push him a bit further: "Well, Sam, maybe nothing will come of this. But if you're willing, I'd like you to go ahead with speaking to someone here as if she were your wife. You might become more aware of feelings you haven't looked at if you try doing this."

Working with a client like Sam can be one of the most difficult tasks a leader faces. He can easily become the target of group hostility, but that hostility will probably do nothing more than increase his defensiveness. In this situation, it is necessary for Peggy to exercise vigilance to prevent him from being attacked. If Peggy were insecure about her abilities, she might use Sam as an excuse to forget her responsibility to the rest of the group and might blame herself for his resistance.

Working with Challenges to Leaders

One of the characteristics of the transition stage is the increased willingness of members to begin to confront the leader, which can often help pave the way for progressing into the working stage. Initially, the members may politely let much of what the leader says go by, without much reaction. If members do have negative reactions to the leader early in the group, they frequently hide them. As the group progresses, members generally show more willingness to express some of the things they have been thinking and internally rehearsing. Indeed, the challenge to leadership can free up members to feel safe enough to begin to confront one another more readily.

How this challenge is dealt with is crucial to the future of the group. If leaders are excessively defensive and refuse to acknowledge criticism, they inhibit the members from confronting one another, with a resulting deleterious effect on the level of trust within the group. In essence, such leaders have established a double standard, one set of norms for intermember confrontation and another set for leader confrontation.

Challenges to leaders are rarely without some foundation in reality. Even though there may be symbolic value or an element of transference in such feedback, at this juncture it may be best for leaders to take the feedback at face value. Leaders who are too quick to interpret such feedback as projection or transference run the risk of closing off the critical member and teaching the group to be excessively cautious about confronting. The ultimate goal, of course, is that members learn that their reactions to others can teach them a great deal about themselves, but at this stage they should simply be encouraged to trust their feelings enough to express them. The leader may want to make a mental note to return at some other time to the possible historical context of the feedback.

Leaders can expect to receive some accurate perceptions both of their role as leaders ("When Mary Ellen cried this morning, you left her hanging." "Why do you let all this attacking go on?") and of their personal characteristics ("You're cold and distant." "You're very authoritarian."). With respect to their role, they need not apologize excessively for it or defend it. Leaders need to explore what members say to them. They can ask questions such as: "What is it that I do that you see as cold and distant?" "What actions do you see as attacking?" What do you wish I had done for Mary Ellen so she wouldn't have been left hanging?" We want to emphasize that in this situation the same rules apply to the leader as to the members. This is an opportunity to model self-disclosure and willingness to listen to feedback. Leaders should not abdicate their leadership responsibilities by making token disclosures, by insisting that they are "just another member," or by embarking on an endless analysis of their characters.

"Why do we always have to focus on the negative?" Roz brings up the issue of her impatience with the group co-leaders, whom she sees as expecting the members to come up with deep problems all the time. She continues by saying: "We always have to have some problem to talk about. There's so much focus on pain in here. I don't see what stops us from talking about some positive things. I get depressed every time I leave this group, and, besides, I'm tired of listening to everyone's problems. I feel pressured by the leaders to always have some burning issue to bring in here."

Before deciding on a technique to use here, the leaders can attempt to discover what Roz means when she says that there is too much focus on the negative. They can ask her to talk more about the pressure she feels from them to have a "burning issue." They might ask her why she is coming to the group if it is not to get some clarity and learn better ways for dealing with areas that present some measure of difficulty for her. Here are some possible meanings of her concern over focusing on the negative:

- Roz may have learned to deal with conflict by avoiding it. When conflict surfaces in the group, she gets uncomfortable and attempts to do what she typically does in everyday life: avoid issues or attempt to smooth things over.
- She may have a lot of pain that she is afraid to acknowledge. Having other members talk about their pain triggers her own anxiety, so she'd rather they focus on pleasant topics.
- Perhaps she is afraid of her depression. She may fear that if she allows herself to feel depressed, she will sink so deeply into a pit she won't be able to pull herself out. Thus, she would rather talk of positive things that won't lead to depression.
- Roz may have "problem envy" and fear that her own struggles, which seem less pressing than those of the others, won't be welcome.
- She may be afraid of anger. For example, she may have experienced considerable anxiety when another member directed anger at her. Or perhaps simply observing others being angry scares her.

All these possible meanings involve fears and resistance; techniques for working with them can be adapted from the examples described in the previous section.

If, however, Roz exhibited much feeling when she said that the leaders expected members to come up with problems all the time, they might introduce a technique for working with her projections. One technique is to ask her to become one of the leaders. In taking this role, she can talk to the group and tell them how they should act in the group.

Once Roz's projections and expectations are out in the open, she can work on some of them. For example, one of the leaders might say to her: "In some ways you seem to see us as responsible for the negative feelings in the group, for after all we are the ones who are focusing on these feelings. We could point the group in a different direction and avoid this focus. Do you want to go further with some of the directions you'd rather see this group take and what you'd want us to do differently?" If Roz says yes, she can say what she fears about each member and how she'd rather see that person act so that she would feel comfortable. She might tell Barbara to cheer up and count her blessings instead of dwelling on her misery. She might tell Bob not to get angry, because his anger scares her. Again, the leaders can be listening for clues of where to go next with Roz. She may attempt to smooth things over in the group and focus on pleasant matters because she had the role of peacemaker in her family. If she would like to change this behavior, the leaders can then introduce techniques that encourage her to do so.

If the trust level is becoming established, the leaders might ask Roz to tell those who have delved into their problems how tired she is of listening to them. She could address these members one at a time and let them know how their work has been affecting her. This could be a powerful catalyst for both her and the others in the group she addresses. They have probably sensed her reactions, and this may be inhibiting them from further discussing their problems. The other members may be fearing judgment or criticism from her, and this technique will probably bring these reactions to the surface. As a result of talking to those members that she is most tired of hearing from, Roz may uncover some of her dynamics. It could be that she is attempting to avoid facing these very problems. It may also be that these people symbolize someone with whom she has a strained relationship. Again, she could accept the challenge to do some further work, if she has decided that it is OK for her to have problems and to work on them in the group.

An alternative strategy for working with Roz is to ask her to complete sentences such as the following:

- "When people in my life express negative thoughts or feelings, I . . ."
- "If only the leaders would . . ."
- "This reminds me of . . ."

This sentence-completion technique is designed to expose her reinforcement history and what she has learned from negative experiences throughout her life. The technique can elicit material for further exploration.

"You leaders aren't sharing enough of yourselves." This sort of remark can be a healthy sign in a group, because it indicates that members are perceiving an inequality—namely, that the leaders are different from all the others in the group in that they don't say much about themselves. At this point the leaders can abdicate their role if they throw out some tidbit about themselves to placate the group. Instead, they might indicate that they are in the group not for their own therapy, as are the members, but to be leaders. They can, of course, share feelings and thoughts concerning the members individually and as a group and acknowledge being touched by personal issues. But generally they can take up these issues with their own therapists.

Also, leaders do not have to apologize for their role. The group is getting to know them through the way they pay attention to members. Leaders become transparent in many ways without talking about personal problems. In other words, they do a disservice to themselves if they have to prove that they, too, are human. It is simply a fact that the group counselor does have a different purpose for being in the group. Leaders make a mistake if they become intimidated by their different role, and it is important that they do not apologize for this difference. But they must explore what the member means by "sharing enough of yourselves." The tone in which they respond to members who want more disclosure is crucial. Either they can convey nondefensiveness and a willingness to reflect about what is being said, or they can respond in a sharp and critical manner that conveys a sense of superiority. Leaders do not have to give the impression that they have arrived and are now "actualized beings." They can let members know that they are still struggling with issues in their own lives but that they do not think it appropriate to pursue these issues in the groups they are leading.

Leaders might examine the motives of members who ask them to show more of themselves. These members are often the same people who become angry with leaders for taking up group time with personal problems or who become condescending after leaders share an issue of their own, such as a feeling of inadequacy. Often such a challenge is based on the members' need to relieve their own anxiety, to have some of the pressure taken off, or to bring the leaders down and make them less intimidating.

Some leaders may feel comfortable sharing not only present reactions but old feelings that come to the surface because of someone else's work. This material can be a catalyst for further group work. Leaders should not display these feelings, however, simply because group members want them to. They may find that attuning themselves to their feelings, both those that arise in the present context and those nurtured through reminiscing about their past, is actually their best tool for listening to others. They may want to spend some time before a group session and during breaks reviewing past and present concerns in their own lives.

Other leaders may be less interested in getting in touch with their own feelings as a prerequisite for leading. If the feelings are there or if they come up within the course of a group, they may express them, but they don't feel the need to stir them up. Some leaders also may not be able to switch in and out of their own intense feelings fast enough to keep their primary focus on the client, to be fully with the group member's work rather than their own. If a personal issue interferes with being with the client, leaders may work on it in the group but only in order to get clear enough to continue work with the client. It is important, however, for leaders to bring into the group any persistent feelings they have that stand in the way of their being able to work with a client. For example, if a leader feels anger, boredom, or annoyance toward a client, the leader may not immediately share these feelings. However, if these feelings persist and get in the way of working with the client, the leader eventually will need to disclose them so that they do not interfere with the relationship between leader and client. If leaders are trying to teach members that feelings are all right, one of the best teaching aids they have is to express feelings themselves.

The main point here is that leaders should not be working on their own material in the group at the expense of the client. If a member brings up a fear of being inadequate, leaders can mention similar concerns of their own in a way that encourages the member to go further. But if the whole group stops so that leaders get to talk about their feelings of inadequacy, the purpose of the group has been lost, and the role of the leader is blurred. If leaders are involved in their own growth, as they should be, they will find that most personal matters can be postponed for discussion with their own therapists.

"You leaders aren't doing your job right." This challenge can take many forms. Members may say that leaders "don't really care for us," "are against us," "are directing us too much," "aren't directing us enough," "aren't getting us started," "are pushing people too much," "leave people hanging,"

"focus too much on pain and hurt," "are using this group to fulfill your own needs," "don't really know what you're doing," or "seem to have a lot of hangups, so how can you lead us?" One technique is to say: "Well, time's up for today. See you next week!"

More seriously, this challenge can be seen as a healthy signal that a group is becoming autonomous. In this situation, you cannot become defensive. You cannot simply dismiss such confrontations as a stage the group is going through, nor can you too readily assume that you are failing. You might ask the members: "What am I not giving you? What are you wanting from me that you're not getting?" Or you might say: "Tell me more. What am I doing or not doing that you don't like?" As members respond, what is important is that you listen and avoid reacting too quickly and in a defensive manner. After they respond and you have taken in what was said, you can then share your reactions about what you heard and how it affected you. In this way you are dealing with your thoughts and feelings as they pertain to what is occurring within the group. At a moment like this, you can model the behavior you hope the group members will learn, including a willingness to explore matters that might trigger a defensive posture.

Another technique is to ask group members how they would like things to be different, if indeed they would, and then to say whether you, as a leader, are willing to do what the members want and why. For example, members may say that they want you to introduce techniques when they feel stuck or when there are long silences. You might reply that you do not want to take on total responsibility for the direction of the group and that you hope that the members will accept their share of the responsibility for what gets accomplished. This technique allows members to clarify what they want and allows you to discuss your own views openly. In fact, you might respond initially to a challenge by saying what you would like to see going on in the group.

In the techniques suggested so far, you are seeking to acknowledge the true parts of the challenge. Of course, you can also explore the possibility of projections. Complaints are often more important for what they say about the members than what they say about the leaders. If you have modeled receptiveness and an ability for handling situations in which you feel defensive, you are in a good position to ask group members to explore the part of themselves that finds fault with others.

"You guys blew it." Every novice group leader worries about making mistakes. In one sense, any input you give as a leader can provide material worth exploring. Regardless of whether members think you are marvelous or a flop, the way they respond can teach them much about themselves. And, although you are still going to worry about being good and effective, you will function better once you begin to worry less, because you then free up your spontaneity and intuition. For all that, all leaders have moments that qualify as mistakes—interventions they regretted, techniques they would have preferred to use differently. Mistakes occur when leaders impose their own agenda rather than being sufficiently ready to follow and flow with the client.

The most economical and appropriate way to handle a misdirected technique is to admit the mistake. We've rarely felt that we lost the respect of our clients when we admitted our mistakes but have found that troubles multiply if we are unwilling to admit mistakes and try to forge ahead. It's a perfect opportunity to model making such an admission without undue defensiveness or remorse. Usually, the emotional momentum that may have been dissipated by the inappropriate intervention can be recovered after such an admission. Sometimes it can't, but the issue that was lost may come up again. The important points here are that you should not hide behind your role or assume you must be perfect and that you should not try to cover up a mistake by imposing yet another technique. As long as you are not trying to hide behind your techniques, it may sometimes be productive to create a technique for constructively exploring your group's reaction once you've gone wrong.

Here are some mistakes that we've made as group practitioners:

- We have given instructions that were too elaborate, complicated, or obscure.
- We have been too hasty in introducing a technique when we were not clear enough about what our members were saying or where we wanted to go with them.
- We have not been sufficiently sensitive to a member's resistance to going along with a technique.
- We have pursued too rigidly an outcome we expected a technique to have and have not been sufficiently tuned in to where a participant was leading us.
- Our interjection of humor has been out of tune with a member's seriousness.
- We have lost the momentum of work in progress by taking too much time setting up a technique or looking for props.
- We have timed techniques poorly, usually because we were not sensitive enough to the member's own pace and were too fixed on our own interpretations or hopes concerning the individual.
- We have set up role-playing situations in which we asked people to take parts that we forgot would be painfully inappropriate for them.
- We have introduced techniques for generating material when we were insufficiently attuned to hidden agendas and issues already present in the group.
- We have had techniques and catalysts in mind for a session and have failed to realize we had too much planned or have failed to be sufficiently attuned to the issues and moods our members brought with them.
- After being threatened, we have become defensive and have been less therapeutic than we might have been.
- We have failed to respond in a personal way to a member who deserved a personal reaction.
- We have introduced an icebreaker technique to get things going when there was no need for it, because the group was already prepared to work.

Concluding Comments

During the transition stage of a group, the following are key tasks for the leader: to continue building trust and cohesion in the group; to continue to invite members to recognize and deal with their fears, anxieties, and hesitations; to be aware of negative reactions and conflict within the group; to point out the value of recognizing and dealing with intermember conflict; to model nondefensive behavior when challenged; to work toward decreasing the dependence of members on the leader and increasing individual responsibility; to encourage members to express persistent feelings about the group; to help members learn how to recognize their ways of avoiding and to teach them ways of challenging their resistances; to teach members directness and effective confrontation; and to enable members to decide on ways in which they are willing to be different in the group.

We conclude this section with some guidelines for effective confrontation. For both members and leaders alike, confrontation is a delicate matter that all too often is handled without sufficient skill and sensitivity. Unless techniques are presented in a caring manner, they are likely to be ineffective in getting participants to recognize and deal with their resistance. One of the functions of a leader is to model constructive confrontation for members and to teach them how to confront one another in an honest and sensitive manner. Below are a few guidelines that you may want to apply to yourself:

- Confrontation is based on the assumption that you care about the person being confronted. It may be helpful for you to imagine yourself as the recipient of the confrontation you are delivering.
- If you are confronting a person, it is a good idea to make a statement about yourself by letting that individual know your purpose in confronting him or her. You might say "Your opinion matters to me, and I wish you would talk more in this group."
- In confronting others, speak primarily about yourself and how you are affected by what they are doing or saying in the group. It may be more accurate to say "I am having a great deal of difficulty in talking to you about this matter" than to say "You are impossible to talk to about this matter." The latter statement is bound to promote defensiveness.
- In confronting people, describe what you see them doing, and avoid labeling them or judging them. It is not helpful to tell a person that he or she talks too much and is a monopolizer. A more effective confrontation is "I want to listen to you and understand you, but I sometimes get lost in your words and don't know what you really want me to hear."
- Confront in a way that encourages others to continue behaving in the way you would like to see them act. Chances are that a person will be put off if you say "You never talk, and it's about time you opened your mouth in here." But they may be helped to express themselves if you say "I really like it when you talk, and I learn a lot from you."

- Be sensitive to the timing of your confrontation. For example, don't confront a member on insufficient participation at a moment when he or she is talking. Instead, reinforce the individual's attempts at making a change.

Questions and Activities

1. How would you describe the characteristics of groups in their transition stage? What do you see as your main tasks as a leader at this stage?
2. How would you work with a member who rejects all attempts to work through resistance? How would your strategy be influenced by whether the group was voluntary or involuntary?
3. Imagine you are a member of a group. What behaviors of yours would constitute resistance? In what specific ways would you resist? What techniques would be especially effective or ineffective in encouraging you to work through your resistance?
4. What are some of your thoughts about questioning as a technique? What difference do you see between closed questions and open questions?
5. Your group members question one another incessantly. What type of technique could you introduce here?
6. Several members of a group you are leading are imposing self-limiting labels ("monopolizer," "the fragile one," "group nurse") at the outset of the group. How might you intervene?
7. What criteria can you use to determine whether a group member whom you consider difficult is actually behaving counterproductively in the group or whether this member is evoking some of your unresolved personal issues?
8. What general guidelines can you come up with for dealing effectively with group members who exhibit problematic behaviors?
9. You have a group member who draws attention to himself in numerous ways. He uses attention-getting behavior whenever the focus is not on him for any length of time, and when attention does center on him, he talks at length, boring or irritating others in the group. Can you think of any techniques for such a situation?
10. Fred is typically sarcastic and hostile. He stops the work of others with his indirect remarks. You sense that the trust level is being lowered by his manner of venting his anger. How would you handle this situation? What might you do about the other members' reactions to him?
11. Sandy typically tells others how they should be, and she is quick to provide solutions to their problems. While aborting their work she also keeps the focus off herself. Can you think of any techniques that you might use in this situation?
12. Imagine how group members might become hostile toward Sam when he says that he can't identify with anyone in the group. Describe some possible techniques for working with this situation. If Sam made his remarks at a preliminary session, would you be likely to include him in or exclude him from the group, and why?

13. Your group members say they are stuck and getting nowhere. What are your thoughts about their complaint and about your responsibility for getting them moving?

14. In the section of this chapter that deals with members' complaining that they are stuck, look at our comments on the various roles that leaders may play, and explain your own views on these roles.

15. Jill comments on not feeling safe in her group. If you were a member in a group, what would it require to make you feel safe in it? How might a leader best work with you on this topic?

16. As Roz comments, groups can often be seen as focusing on negative emotions. If she were to challenge you on this issue, how would you respond? How might you get input from people who had expressed a strong emotion such as sadness or anger in your group? How might your own views on this issue affect the way you work in the group?

17. Look over the list of difficult members in this chapter and think of others whom you might find difficult. Which one pattern of problem behavior do you think you would have the most trouble with? Speculate about the personal dynamics that might be involved in your reactions to this behavior.

18. Some conflicts and struggles for power are inevitable in a group. How do you think techniques can be used in working with conflict? Do you think that conflict can have therapeutic value in a group? Explain.

19. At the fifth meeting, a member who has been relatively silent finally confronts you with his lack of trust in your leadership ability. How might you deal with this challenge?

20. In a group you are leading, a considerable amount of intermember conflict is expressed in several sessions. Finally, a timid and quiet man asks you: "Why are you allowing all this conflict and bickering to take place? What good is all of this doing anybody?" What might you say, and where might you be inclined to go from there?

21. What techniques can you think of to get members to see connections between the sessions? How might you help them work outside the group and bring their results back to a following session?

22. There are many meanings underlying most forms of resistance. How could you facilitate a member's exploration of the meaning of some defensive behavior that you might find annoying?

23. Consider the pattern of behavior that you typically model as a group leader. What kind of group might you have if all of the members in it displayed the behavior that you model?

24. What are some of the ways in which you would explore a client's cultural background as a way of understanding his or her difficult behavior?

25. How would you go about evaluating your own effectiveness as a leader, especially when your group seemed to be experiencing rough times? How would you assess your degree of responsibility as well as the members' responsibility if the group seemed stuck?

CHAPTER SIX

Techniques for the Working Stage

Characteristics of the Working Stage

In this chapter we concentrate on some typical remarks that members might make during the working stage of a group, selecting a phrase or a sentence that seems to especially fit a client. Some of these remarks are rather common, but of course they won't necessarily arise in every group, nor will they always seem important. Different leaders might work with these statements in different ways.

Removed from their context, these remarks by clients may not strike a counselor as profound or promising. Yet given the context of work in progress with a group member, they can be excellent springboards for introducing techniques to pursue a leader's hunch. The statements that a leader picks out often reflect the leader's energy and interests as well as the client's. When we work with a statement, we do not know in advance exactly where it will lead. As often as not, an exercise may develop in an unanticipated direction. The objective is to find ways of bringing issues and feelings into focus, and the statements we discuss here have the promise of helping achieve this objective.

We want to emphasize again that leaders must be willing to abandon a technique and follow whatever material seems to be immediate. We introduce techniques, but clients let us know what direction to pursue. We rarely enter a group with a set idea of the techniques we are going to use. Instead, we invent these techniques during the session, basing them on promising clues and introducing them in such a way as to lead a client into the exercise gracefully and quickly. When a client is already showing some emotion, it is obviously distracting to spend a great deal of time setting up a technique. This sensitivity and spontaneity must be acquired through practice and supervision and cannot be taught in a book.

An underlying rationale for most of the techniques we suggest is that it is not the leader's role to make people feel good or to solve their problems. People must work out for themselves the solutions to the problems they face. However, leaders can provide a setting in which members, through intensifying their thoughts and feelings and sorting them out, can reach a better position to make changes. Quick reassurance and advice do not facilitate self-examination, but respect and a willingness to listen can encourage members to explore issues. Techniques can work simultaneously to intensify experiences and to generate information about the scope of the issue. They can provide clients with the opportunity to express their concerns (which they may be deprived of in everyday life) and to discover connections between present and past experiences in their lives.

During the working stage, we focus on linking members by looking for and pursuing common themes within the group. Leaders should be alert to opportunities for bringing other group members into the work of an individual client. Often part of the reason for picking a specific statement to use in devising a technique is that it seems a promising avenue for including other group members. One of the marks that a group has reached the working stage is the members' ability to spontaneously bring themselves into one another's work. A working group involves a level of cohesion that allows for two or more individuals to work simultaneously on common issues, as opposed to members' taking turns by doing their individual work in a group setting.

A characteristic of the working stage is that participants are usually, although not always, eager to initiate work or bring up themes they want to explore. They do not come to the group saying "Well, I don't know what I want to talk about tonight; I thought I'd go with whatever comes up for me." Sometimes a member's being open to dealing with emerging reactions is fine, for it can lead to some productive work. Yet the person who says "I don't know what I want from this session" is often reflecting a passive stance. There are probably several members in a working group who are clear about what they want, and they are willing to ask for group time. The leader may begin a session with a simple "Who wants to work?" and find that several members declare that they want some time.

This stage is also characterized by a here-and-now focus. A sign of a productive group is that members have learned to talk about what they are currently feeling and doing. Hence, typically their work has a direct quality, rather than a detached storytelling style. Even though members may be exploring problems they have with people outside of the group, they can do their work by dealing with their present feelings and thoughts about these problems. They can also bring problems from their past into the present by working symbolically with significant people in their lives as if those people were present in the room. While an individual is working on outside issues, the leader can also pay attention to what is occurring with other members. By this time, members typically reveal how they are being affected by an individual's work. Again, the group has progressed beyond politely waiting until an individual's work is finished. Members have learned that they can enhance another's work by spontaneously expressing ways in which they are identifying with that person's struggle.

Members are also willing to have direct and meaningful interactions with one another, including confrontations. Conflict in the group is recognized, and members have learned that they need not run away from it. Members are not likely to suppress their feelings of conflict with one another simply because this difficulty is not always immediately resolved. This behavior is quite different from what many of them have learned in their outside lives, where they have demonstrated an "allergic reaction" to sticking with interpersonal conflicts until they are worked through. For instance, if Valerie were to say to Fritz "I wish you weren't in the group, because I don't like you," this comment certainly would not go by unaddressed (at least in our groups). Valerie would be asked to say directly to Fritz more about what she does not like about him and what led up to the conclusions she has formulated about him. She would be challenged to deal with her reactions to him, and he would be given a chance to deal with her, which could open up productive material for both of them. A working group reflects a commitment of people to stay with others through difficult times until all sides have a chance to be given expression. Conflict is not swept under the carpet but becomes the focus for work. How people work through their conflicts in the group situation (or how they avoid doing so) offers many lessons for participants about the sources of their interpersonal problems.

Other characteristics differentiate the working stage from the initial and the transition stages. Members more readily identify their goals and concerns, and they have learned to take responsibility for them. They are less confused about what the group and the leaders expect of them. Most of the participants feel included in the group, or if some do not, they can talk about it in the group. Participants trust the leader's interpretations and suggestions and are less cautious about going along with proposed techniques. Communication in the group is characterized by a free give-and-take among the members and a tendency for them to engage in direct exchanges rather than communicating by way of the leader. The group becomes like an orchestra, in that individual members listen to one another and do productive work together while looking to the conductor for cues.

Members are also more in touch with themselves. They trust themselves more and are more ready to speak their minds, to experiment with different behaviors, and to push themselves to explore personal issues that they find frightening. They are hopeful about the potential for meaningful gain from their participation, and they take more responsibility not only for what goes on within the group but also for carrying what they are learning into their outside lives. They commonly engage in work involving the expression of intense emotion and are not as frightened by it because they have had a chance to see such emotions expressed in constructive ways. They are less concerned about whether they will be accepted for what they say, having seen the group accept people who have shared hidden parts of themselves. Self-disclosure is the norm and is seen as appropriate. There is less game playing and less testing. The members are willing to try to integrate thinking, feeling, and behaving in their everyday life. Issues of transference between members and the leader come out in the open more readily, and members are used to seeing how this transference can teach them about their past and present experiences outside the group.

Intermember exchanges during the working stage are characterized by a giving and receiving of honest, direct, caring, and useful feedback. Members tend to be more trusting of the suggestions they receive, for they now know that people who give them feedback are also willing to receive it.

Group cohesion increases during the working phase. The members have worked together to develop a trusting community, and they respect and care for one another. This sense of community encourages members to explore themselves on a deeper level than is typically true in the beginning stages of the group. The group has earned a level of cohesion through the process of sharing pain, the pain that unites them in their common human experience of struggling. Members who are different in many respects have also found common ground that allows them to take significant risks with one another.

This cohesion is not a static entity, however, and like trust, it tends to ebb and flow. After a very intense session in which powerful work has been done, the members are sometimes frightened by the feelings that have been generated. They may temporarily become more distant, and it may look as though the level of cohesion is waning.

Having said all of this, we also want to point out that the working stage is not always characterized by catharsis and a deeper exploration of issues. In some groups there is likely to be an absence of intense emotions, yet the group can still be functioning well and achieving its goals. In task groups, psychoeducational groups, guidance groups, structured groups, and theme-oriented groups, for example, the participants can be talking honestly, there can be a sense of immediacy, and there can be meaningful interchanges. These clients may show a willingness to cooperate in working on a common agenda, and they may be very committed to the group. They may also demonstrate a willingness to express their differences openly and to struggle with one another to get to the place they would like to reach as a group. In some working groups there may never be a high level of emotional intensity, yet there can still be an honest exchange between members. The interactions may focus on more subtle and seemingly less dramatic issues, but the key point is that the group is characterized by a willingness to work through material rather than shelving issues.

Not all groups reach the stage that we are describing, but that does not necessarily mean that the leader is ineffective. Other factors can keep the group from going beyond the initial stage. Variable membership in a group can inhibit attaining the working stage, particularly if there is no stable core of a few members. Some populations may simply never be ready for the level of intensity we have described. For groups to develop emotional intensity, a therapeutic climate must have been established earlier that makes it possible to engage in a deeper level of risking and personal sharing. Some groups have not established a safe climate, because the members have not yet committed themselves to the demanding work required of a productive group. For example, the participants may simply be showing up and putting in time in the group because they are expected to attend. In addition, if the initial stage is poorly done, the working stage may never be reached. Some groups don't get beyond the unspoken conflicts or fears that inhibited them in their first sessions. The members may be unwilling to give of themselves beyond what is necessary for superficial encounters. They may have collectively decided to stop at a safe and supportive level of interaction rather than to challenge one another to move into unknown territory. Early interchanges between members and the leader or among the members may have been characterized by harsh and uncaring words or actions. The resulting climate of distrust does not encourage members to take the risks necessary to move to a deeper level of interaction. The group may see itself as a problem-solving group—one that discourages full expression of thoughts, beliefs, feelings, attitudes, and experiences. This problem-solving orientation tends to cut off self-exploration, for as soon as a member raises a problem, the other members look for immediate answers. For these reasons and others, some groups never progress beyond the initial stage.

When a group does get to the working stage, it doesn't progress as neatly and tidily as our characterization may suggest. As our comments on the sample statements that follow show, earlier themes of trust, nonconstructive conflict, and reluctance to participate surface again and again. As the group faces new challenges, deeper levels of trust have to be earned. Also, considerable conflict may be resolved in the initial stage, but new conflicts emerge and must be faced. In a sense, a group is like any intimate relationship: it is not static, perfection is never reached, smooth waters may turn into stormy waters for a time, and commitment is necessary to do the difficult yet rewarding work of moving forward.

Working with Emerging Themes

In this section we present a variety of themes that might emerge in a working group. Our intention is to give some flavor of the struggles that individuals bring to the sessions and to demonstrate possible techniques in helping members explore their concerns in more depth. As will become evident, some of the following statements sound like ones that could be made during the transition period in a group's development. In the working stage, however, the members show a willingness to go beyond the point at which they have typically stopped because of anxiety. Their commitment to work often has the effect of triggering other members, which can easily lead to the development of common themes that unite the group.

"I'm confused and don't know what to do." A statement expressing confusion can sometimes be a form of unconscious resistance. It may come from children of rigid and authoritarian parents. In some fashion the therapist is seen as a parent trying to get the client to do some work.

We might begin by asking Betty to say more about what she is confused about. Often, confusion represents a pulling in different directions and prevents the person from taking a stand one way or the other. To accentuate these polarities and to provide Betty with a means of gathering more data so that she can clarify which direction she wants to take, we can include other members by asking them to take sides. For instance, if she has a dual urge to move closer to people and also to pull back as soon as she begins to approach them, some members can try to persuade her of the advantages of intimacy. Other members can take the opposite position and urge her to pull back, stressing the disadvantages of getting close to others. During this time she remains silent and allows herself to go toward each position. Then she can talk about what she experienced as she allowed herself to go back and forth. This technique is likely to touch other members who are struggling with similar choices, and these members can then talk to one another about their conflicts. In this way, the work of several members can be linked.

Another technique consists of having Betty follow her intuitions, even if she is confused. The rationale here is to deal with her resistance by following her energy and the leads that she does give us. After she says she is confused, the leader says "What is it that you feel like doing now?" She replies "I want to pull back." The leader says: "OK, pull back. Go back behind the sofa, and when you feel like saying anything, say it." The leader then continues with whoever in the group wants to speak. After a while Betty rises to her knees and peers from over the back of the sofa. The leader asks "Is there something you would like to say?" Betty replies "No, I just want to stay here." The leader allows her to do so by saying "That's fine, but whenever you want to say something, let us know." In a few minutes she breaks in and says "I want to come back in." Once she has done so, the leader says "Now that you're in, is there anything you want to say or do?" She says she would like to sit between Al and Pete and have them close to her. The leader continues "Now what would you like to do?" She replies "I would like to lean against Pete." The leader asks her what she would like to say to Pete. She says "I feel like a little child." "How old are you?" the leader asks. "Twelve." "What would you like to say to Pete now?" At this point Betty needs little assistance, and she is likely to talk about a painful childhood experience involving a parent.

When a client like Betty makes a statement such as "I'm confused," it should be clear to the leader that she is stuck and unable to proceed. Directly confronting her would just entrench the resistance. In agreeing with her and in a sense handing the direction of the work over to her, the leader leaves her with no one to resist. All the leader needs to do is say: "What do you want to do now?" "What do you want to say now?" "Do whatever you want to do." This technique bypasses resistance by having the leader join the client in her resistance and allowing her to lead the way.

Depending on the leader's relationship with Betty, he might prod her with remarks such as: "Pretend you weren't confused. What would you be saying now if you knew what you wanted?" A related technique consists of asking her to act for a week as if she were not confused. She can be given the homework assignment to assume that she is clear and confident. If she responds with: "This sounds like a good assignment, and I'm willing to give it a try, but I'm afraid I'll feel even more confused in spite of trying to convince myself that I'm clear. Then what do I do?" The leader could respond with: "Well, are you willing to go about your business, even if you're confused, but still tell yourself that you might just know what you want and then act this way?" Another strategy would be to ask Betty to make an alliance with someone in the group and to call that person to report on how this assignment is going. All these techniques put increased responsibility on her to do something cognitively and behaviorally outside of the group meetings to move beyond the place where she typically gets stuck. Of course, she can bring back to the following session a report of what she learned by carrying out this assignment.

There is yet another technique to use when Betty says that she is confused. The leader can reply with: "Whom in this group would you want to get closer to right now? Are you willing to go to that person and talk to him or her about why you want to get close?" Betty may be very unclear initially about why she is drawn to a particular person. However, it is not really important that she know why she feels close to this person. She will probably get a lot more clarity if she is willing to take action and go up to a person and initiate this work. The client she picks to talk to might become personally involved in the work, and this could enhance both members' work.

"I'm afraid to get close to people." This example shares some of the dynamics of the previous example of Betty's confusion. Some of the techniques employed with Betty could also be used in the following example with Carl. The leader can begin by asking him whether he wants to explore the issue of closeness. Does he really want to get close? Is it all right with him if he doesn't? Whom does he want to get close to in his life right now? Sometimes it is not clear how genuinely people are involved with issues they introduce. By asking Carl these questions, the leader can allow him to focus on whether this issue is pressing for him or whether he is getting what he wants as things are now.

If, as Carl talks, the leader senses that although this is a significant topic for him, he is not expressing much feeling, she can ask him to talk about the closeness he feels is missing between him and others in the group. Any of these questions could enable him to explore his fear of intimacy within the here-and-now context of the group: "Whom in here might you want to get closer to? And what has stopped you so far?" "How close do you think that people in here feel to you? And what might you be doing to either draw people toward you or push them away from you?" "What are some things that you tell yourself when you imagine yourself developing intimacy with us?" "Is there anything you want to say to anyone in here that you've thought about but haven't said?" This technique brings the rest of the group into Carl's work and provides an opportunity for feedback from others about whether he behaves in ways that keep him from having much intimacy with them. It also picks up on his use of the word *afraid* and gives him an opportunity to discuss what the fears might be. These are some possible implications:

- He may have lost someone important to him either through death or the dissolution of a relationship.
- He may feel that there is something about him that people will not like if they get close enough to be aware of it.
- He may have convinced himself that he has absolutely nothing to give anyone.
- He may feel that intimacy with another will lead to his feeling smothered or trapped.

- He may be afraid that getting close will lead to a sexual encounter.
- He may be hurting over a divorce.
- He may fear too much commitment or too many demands.
- He may be uncomfortable with being accepted or loved.
- He may have had overprotective parents.

If Carl's fears of closeness stem from parental injunctions and tacit communications such as "Don't get close" or "Don't get committed," the leader can pursue the topic by asking questions such as these: What specifically did he hear from his parents or learn nonverbally? Who in his life told him not to be close? Next, he can pretend he is that person and stand up and lecture the members on why they should not get close to anyone. What would this person—perhaps his father—say about his getting close to each member of this group? And what would he want to say in reply to his father? Through this technique he can come to understand how he carries out these parental injunctions by being the way he has been in the group. The leader can continue by getting him to look at early decisions he made, such as "If I don't get close, I won't be rejected" or "I'm not going to be hurt again by being abandoned." The leader can then return to how he currently keeps himself from closeness in the group and in everyday life.

"This isn't the real world." Cheryl brings up an issue that she wants to work on in the group. She is having trouble in applying what she experiences in the group to her life at work and at home. She feels free to disclose her reactions in the group, for she is supported in doing so. She can get angry with someone in the group, say what is provoking her, and work toward a resolution of differences. But she is afraid that if she were to say what she felt on her job, she'd soon be fired. At home, too, she is hesitant to be open with members of her family. She is afraid that they would not listen to her and that they would be hurt by her disclosures. Her basic task is to learn what is appropriate disclosure and how to make such disclosures without making others defensive.

One technique to use here is for the leader to ask Cheryl to describe a particularly difficult situation and to say what she'd like to change in it. She says that she doesn't like the way she responds to her co-workers in the office. She sees herself as extremely careful of what she says to them lest she hurt their feelings and offend them. She constantly censors what she is about to say and attempts to figure out what her co-workers want to hear. She would like to feel free to tell these people what's on her mind, uncensored. After sketching the situation, Cheryl can select several "co-workers" from the group, describe an incident in the office, and tell how she typically would act in this situation. Then, she can try to tell each of the co-workers in the group things she'd not normally say, and she can say aloud what she is thinking and telling herself as she is talking with each of them. This exercise should uncover how she stops herself from being more forthright. She may be seeking approval from a co-worker. Or she may be suppressing her anger over the way she feels treated by that person. She may be intimidated by another's sarcasm and put-downs. The leader can eventually have her focus on one of the co-workers and say more of what she typically censors out. She can at least be encouraged to tell this person how she is feeling in the person's presence. After the role playing, both the members and the leader can provide feedback to Cheryl by telling her how they might feel if they were her co-worker. How willing would they be to listen to her? How were they affected by her?

Through the role-playing exercise Cheryl can learn a lot about the impact she has on others. Perhaps she demands that others be self-disclosing or in some way meet her expectations. Or she may focus on how she'd like them to be different instead of on how she could retain her integrity in spite of the fact that some people around her are not willing or ready to change the way she'd like them to. In short, she can learn how to confront others without increasing their defensiveness. The specific feedback after role playing is helpful to members such as Cheryl who may not be aware of how their style of disclosure puts others off.

The leader may want to point out to Cheryl and the other members that what occurs in a group can be realistic. Members not only can be open and trusting in the group but also can take risks selectively with people on the outside. The key word is *selectively*, for Cheryl can be setting herself up for failure if she attempts to open up with everyone she knows. She needs to decide how important a given relationship is to her. She may well decide, for example, not to tell her boss everything she thinks, for she might indeed put her job in jeopardy by doing so. It is therapeutic for her to say what she typically keeps bottled up inside of her in the supportive atmosphere of the group, but it may be unwise for her to do the same at work. However, she can still recognize within herself what she is feeling, and she does not have to repress those feelings even though she keeps them to herself. From this growth experience, she can also learn to find someone with whom she can talk about feelings that she chooses not to express to her boss.

We frequently focus members on the potential consequences if they said in their everyday life what they sometimes say in role-playing situations in the group. We attempt to teach people how they may not get the results they want if they confront others too directly at work. In a case such as Cheryl's, we would help her examine the consequences that might follow if she decided to confront people in her life. We don't tell her not to confront, but we do help her assess the risks involved and help her decide what she most wants to say and what she might not want to say to others. Through her work in the group, she may discover that some of her reactions toward her boss are the result of transference. Her boss may be getting more than his or her fair share. Part of the group process involves providing members with skills that will lead to bridging the gap between the group and the real world.

"If I started crying, I'm afraid I'd never stop."   Although many people in the group have taken significant risks by opening up deep wounds and allowing themselves to begin a process of healing, a few members have kept themselves in check and consistently dealt with their problems in a more cognitive manner. Jane is one of those members who are aware that they are preventing themselves from experiencing the depth of their feelings. She admits that she has held herself back through much of the group's life. When the leader asks about her behavior, she says she is afraid that if she started to cry, she might never stop. In such a situation, the leader might begin by pointing out that when people show their feelings, these feelings tend to be short-lived, but when they do not permit themselves to cry, they may spend a lifetime being sad. He might add that he has never yet seen anyone in a group cry for more than twenty minutes, perhaps. Having said this, the leader can ask Jane whether she wants to try letting go of her emotional control. If she agrees, the leader can have her sit in front of Sally, whose eyes are still moist from work she was involved in a few minutes before. Keeping eye contact with Sally, Jane can talk about some of the things she holds herself back from crying about. The emotion still evident in Sally's face may serve as a catalyst for evoking feeling in Jane.

Or the leader can ask Jane to tell Sally how she is affected by Sally's tears. Jane may get through her resistance to crying by talking to Sally about her reaction. During this exercise, the leader might suggest any or all of these sentences for Jane to complete as she continues her contact with Sally:

- "I wish you hadn't cried, Sally, because when you did I . . ."
- "If I were to cry like that, I would . . ."
- "If I were to cry, I would cry about . . ."
- "One reason I can't cry is . . ."
- "Tears don't do any good because . . ."
- "The people in my life who cried were . . ."
- "The people in my life who didn't cry were . . ."
- "No matter what you do, Sally, I'll never cry because . . ."

The leader can take cues for further work from Jane's replies. Sally also should respond by saying what it was like for her as Jane talked directly to her. Finally, to connect others in the group to this work, they can be asked to express to either Jane or Sally how they were affected by the interaction.

Although it's preferable to allow clients to supply the material with which they want to work (as in the case of Betty and her confusion), leaders may sometimes want to search for material that they are not sure exists. Suppose Jane is willing but still feels stuck. She is sitting before Sally and seems to have no idea what to say. The leader can try a hunch: "Jane, I wonder whether there has ever been a person in your life over whom you needed to cry, yet you didn't allow yourself to?" The leader formulates a broad question in which almost anyone could find something to pursue. The leader may suspect that Jane is still mourning the death of someone important to her and that her grief contributes to her depressive style. But mentioning death here is too specific and threatening. Instead, the leader gives Jane an opportunity and leaves her enough room to pull back.

"I'm afraid I'll go crazy." Dave expresses his fear that deep down inside he has the potential for going crazy. Apparently, he sees craziness almost as if it were tangible—a thing inside him, like a tumor, that resides there undiagnosed. Assume that Dave is a member of a group composed of relatively well-functioning people. The leader can get him to work with the paradoxical idea that people gain control in their emotional lives when they become willing to lose control, when they give up rigid fears about what they would be like if they did not keep their emotions in check all the time. In doing such work, however, Dave may become so fascinated with acting like a crazy person that the leader is concerned. At this point it may be appropriate for the leader to say: "You know, Dave, there are ways I see you as working very hard at proving that you are crazy. So in spite of the fact that I'm generally encouraging people here to be unrestrained in their expression of feeling, I'd like to encourage you to realize that you could indeed be crazy if you insisted on it. It might be more productive for you to work on not overwhelming yourself." The leader is attempting with this intervention to get Dave to see that he indeed is contributing to his own frenzy by all the things he is telling himself. The leader hopes that she can prevent him from overwhelming himself by taking in too much all at one time. Her intervention is basically geared to slowing him down and helping him become more centered.

In more normal circumstances, the leader might start out by asking Dave a question: "I wonder where you got the idea that you might 'go crazy,' and I wonder what that expression might mean to you?" He may say that there is a history of mental illness in his family. Or he may have been told that masturbating or expressing anger could make people crazy. Next, the leader might invite him and other members who have expressed the same concern to stage a demonstration of how they think they might behave if they were crazy. Instead of staging a demonstration, Dave may say "I think I would just sit here in a stupor and not interact with anyone." Another member may reply "It seems to me, Dave, that this is pretty much what you've been doing in this group." The point here is both to acknowledge Dave's concern and to provide a vehicle for confronting it.

Leaders should keep several points in mind in connection with this example. First, all counselors and group leaders should think through their own theoretical positions about mental illness regardless of whether they work with institutionalized people or relatively well-functioning clients. Our own perspective is that what appears to be "crazy behavior" is at times a way of acting that a client chooses for the purposes of psychological survival. We acknowledge that such behavior is not always a choice. Not all readers will share our theoretical convictions.

Second, leaders must explore their fears of handling a group member who is going crazy and their own fears of going crazy as well. Leaders who are frightened by their own potential for bizarre behavior can easily reinforce the fears of a client working on this problem and of the rest of the group. Those leaders who are uncertain about their own psychological stability would have a difficult time in working with the fears others have of losing control or of acting in crazy ways.

Third, counselors should be cautious in urging clients to go further than they are willing to go themselves. Counselors have no business encouraging clients to travel a path that they themselves have not walked. What is perhaps most frightening to an inexperienced leader conducting a group composed of presumably relatively well-functioning individuals is to find that someone's behavior is fragmented to a degree that the leader finds unsettling. Experienced leaders tend not to be afraid of clients' being or going crazy, and this trust in members is an asset to the work clients are willing and able to do. Among the fears that typically haunt a group, the fear of being crazy is one of the biggest. Here, as elsewhere, the leaders' biggest concern should be for those fears that clients are afraid to express, and leaders can help make the group a place where clients can express and examine those fears.

Fourth, when people have done something in the group that they regard as crazy, it is important for the leader to follow up by establishing contact between them and the group. If this is not done, the person who expressed fears of going crazy is likely to withdraw because of embarrassment and concern over what others might be thinking. Invariably, in these situations we do everything we can to encourage members to talk about what they are telling themselves, including how they think others are judging them. Our techniques are aimed at helping them make contact with others in the room by talking about their feelings of embarrassment or their ambivalence. By doing so, they are more apt to stay present and deal with whatever is going on with them.

Working with Intense Emotions in All Members Simultaneously

In this section we describe how a number of members are sometimes triggered by one another's work and become emotionally involved simultaneously. This can occur when clients allow themselves to reexperience painful memories associated with certain life events. At times, they may feel they will lose control. Such emotional energy can be, depending on the group, productive and positive. This is not a usual phenomenon in most groups, and it should not be used as an index to measure a working group. In other words, the absence of this phenomenon does not signify that the group is unproductive. When such emotional release does occur, however, it is the result of the cohesive and trusting climate that is generally reached during the working phase.

How might you, as a group leader, work with several members who were at once caught up in sobbing and crying? First of all, it is almost impossible to predict just what will trigger these emotional releases. Someone who is affected by another person's work will simply intervene by also expressing an intense emotional reaction. The alert leader can be sensitive to this development by staying attuned not only to the person working but also to others in the group; co-leaders are an asset here. One technique is simply to bring the focus back to just one person: "There seems to be a lot of strong emotion in this room. Maybe we could all try for now to stay with Charlie and what he's dealing with." An alternative is to look for ways to link the work of several members. If you sense that more than one member could benefit from a catharsis at the same time, you can invite several people to sit in the center of the group facing one another and to share their feelings. Others may be added to this inner working circle either at their own initiative or with your prompting. You need to have sufficient trust in this process to allow it to take its own course. Do not be so concerned with keeping the focus on the person who had been working that you short-circuit the emergence of this phenomenon. You should make a mental note to come back to the person who had been in the spotlight when there is an opportunity later.

Once many people have begun expressing their emotions, you have to make a quick decision about which member to work with. You may want to move near or next to a person who is sobbing. At the same time you must glance about the room to keep track of what is going on elsewhere. At this point all the participants are potential resources for one another and can work constructively together. You may, with a word or gesture, pair people up and have them explore together what they are feeling or offer each other comfort and support. You can draw on recollections of which people have previously interacted and of who seems to symbolize what to whom. For example, the woman who typically tries to soothe another's pain and never expresses her own may sob like a baby in someone else's arms. The man who fears being incapable of loving others may cry silently as he lets himself be with and comfort another member.

For various reasons, you may decide that some members are getting lost in their emotionality. The procedures one would ordinarily use to intensify emotional expression can be reversed to help a person gain distance and perspective. For instance, you can intensify a member's work by asking him to talk directly to the person with whom he has an issue. To deintensify the expression of this member, you might say: "Your mother isn't really here right now. I'm here. I'd like for you to look at me and talk with me about the feelings you have just been expressing and about what you want to learn from this work."

It is important to be aware that the catharses that we have described do not last for a long time. Eventually, the group calms down. A glance around the room reveals a lot of moist eyes, a lot of comforting and tenderness, perhaps some laughter, and a few dazed or frightened people who have stayed on the sidelines. As the room begins to come back to normal, you may suggest that the group return to the original seating arrangement. It is then useful to check in with the person whose work provided a catalyst to determine if he or she has any need to take care of unfinished business. You can also encourage both those who became swept up in the event and those who did not to discuss what they were feeling while it was going on. It is important for you to solidify the lesson that should be apparent—that people can allow themselves a period of intense emotional release and be left sane, intact, peaceful, even joyful.

The material that people express during such cathartic sessions can be important and profound, but it is easy soon afterward to forget what one was thinking, feeling, and saying. Therefore, as soon as is feasible, all members can recall aloud the specifics of what they were experiencing and can focus on the insights and feelings they want to remember and learn from.

Working with Dreams

"I had a dream."   Patty reports a portion of a dream that she would like to explore. Here are some ideas for working with her. She can report the dream in the present tense, as if it were taking place now. If she can't remember part of the dream, she can invent the missing part, or "dream it up." As she presents the dream, you can pay attention to her voice, her level of energy, her body posture, and the parts she seems to gloss over as unimportant. At the end of her report, she can say how she felt on awakening, how she felt during the dream, and how she felt while reporting her dream. She can tell what she learned from the dream or how it might tie in with what is going on in her daily life. In short, you can try to get an initial sense of what she might think the dream means. To work on the dream in more detail, Patty can assign different parts of it (persons or things) to various members of the group and coach the members on what they might say in those roles. She can tell each person why she picked him or her for the part and why that member was well suited for it. She can also be each part of the dream herself and carry on a dialogue with the other parts. If she was walking toward a door in her dream, she can be the door and talk to Patty and then be Patty and talk to the door. You can also try to utilize props available in the room. For instance, Patty can have a dialogue with an actual door. She can also construct a different ending for her dream. Then she or others in the group can act this new ending out.

Another technique for working on Patty's dream in detail is to invent sentence completions from the key phrases or concepts in the dream. For example, she can start by saying "If I were a door I would . . ." Or, if she used the word *scared* in reporting the dream, she can complete several versions of the sentence "What scares me most in my life right now is . . ."

To involve other members more directly, you can ask those who seem especially interested to talk about Patty's dream as if it were their own and to act out various parts. Or they can free-associate to what they regard as interesting symbols in the dream. The group members can also argue over and decide which parts of the dream they want to act out according to their own fantasies. The point here is not for them to interpret for Patty but to use her dream as a tool for looking at themselves.

Techniques for working with dreams can be modified or abandoned as other issues or reactions from others in the group begin to surface. Involving other members allows you to use Patty's dream for working with her and others in the group simultaneously. In addition, simply allowing the client to report a dream without elaborate attempts at interpretation is valuable. There may be little necessity for the use of techniques at all.

"I had a dream about the group." During our weeklong residential groups a member sometimes dreams about the group. Melissa had such a dream on the second night: "I am in the back of a big tractor with Patrick [a leader] driving it. The tractor has no trailer attached, just the cab. We are driving through this small town when, suddenly, faceless people stop our cab and start beating on the windows. I cry out to Patrick 'Do something,' and he says 'Don't worry, there's no danger.' I look around and these faceless people seem to be all over the place, attacking people in the town. But then I notice that nobody seems to get hurt and no harm seems to have been done." Even though the meaning seems obvious, Melissa can profit from interpreting the dream in Gestalt fashion.

She can begin by speaking *as Melissa:* "I'm Melissa. I'm in this big tractor with Patrick driving. I feel very safe and happy in here with him driving. I'm going to curl up in the sleeping compartment of this tractor and go to sleep." *As Patrick:* "I'm Patrick. I know what I'm doing. I know where to take this rig, and I feel good about what I'm doing." *As the tractor:* "I'm a great big tractor. I'm strong. I'm made of steel, and I command respect wherever I go. I haul heavy burdens for long periods, and I provide safety to those who ride in my cab." *As the faceless people:* "We are faceless people. We terrify others. They cringe and try to hide from us, and they think we're going to beat them up and kill them." *As Melissa to Patrick:* "Do something. You're the driver. You're supposed to help me. I trusted you, and yet here you are doing nothing to protect us." *As Patrick to Melissa:* "Don't worry. Be patient. You'll see that no harm comes to anybody. You're safe in here, even though it looks dangerous."

Melissa obviously is struggling with trust, both of Patrick's leading and of the group members. The next step is to have her tell the "faceless people" in the group how she sees them as dangerous and attacking. She can also tell Patrick how he is not protecting her.

A suggestion for working with dreams is not to worry too much about what a dream "really means," preferring instead to look for what meaning can be created with the help of dream materials. In that spirit, it is often useful to treat a dream as if it were about the group, without seeking to imply that this is in fact what the dream is all about. For example, after an initial and somewhat sluggish checking in by all the members of an ongoing weekly group, Raphael reports this dream: "I was alone, and for some reason

I was afraid there was going to be this earthquake. And then there was an earthquake of sorts, except that it wasn't any violent shaking or anything like that. There was just this big chasm that started to appear, and where I was sitting was a piece of land that separated from the land on the other side, and it just drifted farther and farther away."

The leader makes a few efforts to draw out further thoughts from Raphael about this dream, but little seems to come to his mind. Eventually the leader proposes this: "You know, Raphael, I really don't have much of a sense of what's going on in your dream, but it does serve to help me express something that's going on in this group. I thought there was some tension here a couple of weeks ago that wasn't really addressed last week, and like the earthquake that never quite happened, I'm thinking there's something that's not happening here tonight." Now Melissa speaks up: "That sure fits for me. I'm feeling as if Janice and I are drifting apart after what we disagreed about a few meetings ago, and now it seems this whole group is afraid of an earthquake." The leader says "I wonder whether anyone here can think of a way to interpret Raphael's dream as a metaphor for describing what we need to be addressing within this group." Raphael says "Well I think we're each going to feel as isolated and alone as I do in this dream if we can't be a bit more honest with the 'earthquakes' we fear having with one another."

Working with Projections and Other Problems of Self-Awareness

"I can't talk to my parents." In response to Dee's complaint about dealing with her parents, we are likely to say: "Let's see whether we can learn more about what makes you feel this way. I'd like you to pick out two people here who you can pretend are your parents. Don't worry about whether there's any real similarity. All you need is two pairs of eyes to look at as you proceed. Now, talk directly to your pretend parents, and tell them a bit of what you find hard to talk to them about." Dee can start off with the sentence "Mom [Dad], it's hard to talk to you because . . ." or "When I try to talk with you, I feel . . ." By talking directly to her pretend parents, Dee mobilizes feelings that she may avoid by merely talking *about* her parents. The exercise thus provides practice in communicating in a direct and honest way. This technique may lead to exploring the content of what Dee won't talk about with her parents, or it may lead to clarifying the process of that communication and how it is inhibited. Thus it provides her with an opportunity both for practicing what she experiences as difficult and for gaining insight into the nature of the difficulty.

Our request that Dee not worry about any real similarity between her actual parents and the pretend parents forestalls her saying that no one in the group is much like her parents. That may be true, but it doesn't provide much to work with, and it bypasses the opportunity for her to get some practice as well as some insight. The pretend parents may turn out to be good substitute parents, and the material they open up can be explored either by her or by the group members who are the pretend parents. Depending on context and hunches, we may want to encourage the pretend parents to respond to Dee. They might let her know how they are affected by the feedback they are getting. Her work could even stimulate feelings in the pretend parents about their own children. In this case, it could be very useful for all involved to continue working in this vein. Initially, it may be best for Dee to get things out in the open without interruption; then, after she has had a chance to express herself to her pretend parents, they can respond. But an emotionally productive and relevant scene may emerge from a dialogue between Dee and her pretend parents, especially if she does some coaching or role swapping. Even inappropriate input from one of the pretend parents can be used to advantage. For instance, "Dad" may do more talking than listening until Dee becomes frustrated enough to say that in real life her father's similar behavior is part of the problem. Almost any material that comes out of such an interaction can be very productive grist for the mill. If the father is the "ideal father" Dee wishes for, she can tell him how it is to have these feelings for him. If the father is one who frustrates her, she can then explore her feelings of not getting what she wants from him. The specific path the work takes is typically determined by the clues the client will provide or ways in which other members may be triggered by one client's work. Again, we facilitate linking among members so that they can make the fullest use of the group process.

"My father wouldn't speak in English." This example illustrates how leaders might work with a person's voice and how they might encourage him to use his native language. Carlos has been given the feedback that he sounds abrasive. There is gentleness in his eyes and in the content of his remarks, but he has a way of using his voice that leaves people feeling under attack. He acknowledges the validity of this feedback and wants to explore the theme further.

Drawing on clues from earlier work, the leader can ask Carlos to think how the voice of each of his parents sounded to him when he was a child and to give imitations of each while saying "I'm reluctant to be gentle because . . ." The leader may have a hunch that in many ways Carlos is reluctant to be like his father, a kindly man much belittled by Carlos's mother. Sure enough, the imitation of his mother comes across as abrasive. When he starts to present an imitation of his father, Carlos remarks "My father wouldn't speak in English."

When we are working with bicultural and bilingual clients, we often take the initiative to ask them what language they speak with their family members and friends. Frequently, the techniques we suggest in these cases involve talking in their native language to a loved one (if this person is a key individual in a problem they are exploring). People often display some resistance when asked to work in their native language. Talking in English can distance these clients, whereas their own language may bring back painful associations. Nevertheless, even though the leader does not speak or understand Carlos's native tongue (Spanish), Carlos is willing to proceed by playing the role of his father talking to his mother about what his kindness has cost him. As Carlos proceeds, the leader can be attentive to clues of emotional intensity and urge him to repeat phrases that seem to bring him closer to his feelings: "Say that again, please." Eventually, Carlos stops after some anger and some crying. By using this technique, the leader demonstrates a willingness to stay with Carlos's emotions even when the content is unknown. The leader can then ask him to review, in English, what his work has taught him. He may say that he is afraid to sound like his father for fear that women will treat him as his father was treated by his mother. He can then try a new voice and say something to each of the women in the group. Other members may comment on how he now seems gentle and yet powerful and attractive. Carlos is not likely to leave the group with a permanent new voice, but he can see the options he has for a different style, and he can acquire considerable insight into how others experience him and the reasons for his abrasiveness.

If other group members have some fluency in the working member's language, we are likely to utilize them. For instance, we might direct Carlos's role-playing remarks to one of them. But it is not essential that anyone be familiar with the language. Many times in using this sort of technique with a person like Carlos, we find that other members are deeply touched by his work even though they don't understand the content of what he is saying. They are able to pick up the general emotional tone through his voice and nonverbal forms of communication. If they are emotionally involved, it is a good practice to ask those members, once Carlos has finished a piece of his work, to tell him how he affected them. This can be powerful feedback for Carlos and for the members who give the feedback as well. It can also be an ideal place to continue the therapeutic work by inviting others whose own issues are surfacing to talk about themselves. Often all that needs to be said is something like: "Joyce, you really seem affected by Carlos. Tell him more about what you are feeling." If Joyce says that this work is bringing up painful issues with her father, the leader could say: "Look around the room, Joyce. Who in here do you see that could be most helpful to you right now? How about picking a pair of eyes and talking to that person as your father. Let your 'father' know about some of that pain that you've been keeping to yourself."

"I feel the burdens of the world." Judy seems so tired, so weary. At an earlier session she was confronted by Jack for being too quick to try to rescue him when he was discussing a conflict of his. She revealed then that during her childhood she often took on the role of the family arbitrator, always seeking to smooth over quarrels between her parents. Today, after completing some work with Jennifer involving a great deal of sadness, Judy looks exhausted. When she is asked what she is feeling, she says "I feel the burdens of the world."

One technique for exploring her feelings is to have her exaggerate them: "Judy, would you be willing to pick up that stack of telephone books [or any heavy object] and hold them while you talk to us about the burdens you feel. I'd like for you to really allow yourself to feel their weight, as you talk, and allow them to symbolize how laden you feel." A bioenergetic technique to accent this burden further is to ask Judy to stand with her knees slightly bent in order to add to the experience of stress.

As Judy lists various burdens she is aware of, the rest of the group can be connected to her work by having her stand before each member, one at a time, still holding the books, and complete the sentence "You burden me by . . .": "Jennifer, you burden me by being so sad. I want you to be happy." "Jack, you burden me with your anger. I want everything to be peaceful." After completing this go-around, Judy can make another round, this time using the sentence "I burden myself by . . .": "Jennifer, I burden myself by worrying so much about your being sad." "Jack, I burden myself by thinking I have to be responsible for solving your conflicts." This technique gives Judy some insight into how she is responsible for the way she takes on other people's burdens.

At one point, standing before Charlene, she says "Mother, I burdened myself by wanting you and Dad to get along better." Here the leader can drop the technique in progress and replace it with one designed to pursue the client's lead: "Judy, why don't you just stay there in front of Charlene and continue to talk with her as if she were your mother. Let's hear more of how you may have burdened yourself as a child."

Eventually, the work may get back to how Judy is burdening herself in the here and now. Because people are often reluctant to give up the things they complain of, the leader might now try a technique designed to facilitate looking at this phenomenon. Judy (who is still holding the telephone books or some other heavy object) can continue on around the circle giving up a burden, and a book, to each group member. After she has completed this exercise and given up her books, the leader can ask her to make a plan of action: "During this coming week, if you find yourself taking on any of the burdens you just relinquished, call one of the members of the group, whoever would be most appropriate, and ask to have the burden back." As an adjunct to carrying out this plan, Judy could be asked to spend some time writing in her journal about what she got from this work in the session. She might write her mother an uncensored letter, which she does not mail, as a way to further express some of her feelings that have been tapped in this session. This would be a good time to ask Judy what she might come up with by way of additional homework assignments that she could practice during the week. This strategy keeps the focus of responsibility on Judy for deciding on the ways in which she wants to change and for taking concrete steps to bring these changes about.

In work such as that between Judy and her "mother," leaders might be alert for ways to bring other members into the flow of work. For example, Judy is talking to a member as her mother about all the ways in which she feels burdened by her. It is very possible that the person sitting in for Mother (Charlene) is touched by her own concerns. She may be strongly identifying with Judy. Or she may be very much identifying with the mother and may be resenting what she is hearing from Judy. There may well be other members who are deeply touched by the role playing, and it could be most helpful to bring them into the work. There is no reason why the leader needs to work exclusively with Judy and ignore others' issues that surface. There is therapeutic potential in asking Judy and Charlene to do their own work with each other. If the leader is successful in bringing other members to do their own work by responding to Judy or Charlene, this can very well accelerate both women's work. From our perspective, groups are functioning at their best not when we are doing individual therapy with others observing but when we are able to effectively bring in several other people with related themes. Then we are making the best use of the group process as a learning mechanism.

The leader in this example draws on several modalities: Gestalt therapy, in asking Judy to exaggerate and in bypassing resistance by the use of incomplete sentences; bioenergetics, in having Judy bend her knees and experience her stress fully on a physical level; psychoanalysis, in focusing on resistance and then insight; and behavior therapy and reality therapy, in asking Judy to make an action plan and giving her homework assignments. The work in this example thus touches the three areas of thinking, feeling, and doing.

"Here, let me help all of you." Although not explicitly stated, Claude's underlying attitude seems to be "Let me help all of you." I know how you feel, because I was once there myself. I've got the answer for you." This attitude cuts off exploration. Although it is important for leaders not to ridicule a helping attitude, they need to distinguish between facilitative and non-facilitative helpfulness. If Claude's nonfacilitative helpfulness is not dealt with, the group will slow down. It may be valuable to bring his attitude into focus by introducing a way of exploring it. For instance, the leader might say: "Claude, I notice that you seem ready to come to the assistance of people, and yet I very rarely hear you asking for any help for yourself. I remember your saying at the beginning of the group that you were burned out on giving to your family, because you got so little in return. It may be that you're behaving in this group in many of the ways you do outside of here. Would you be willing to explore this?" If Claude agrees, the leader can suggest one of these go-arounds:

- "Go around to each person in the group and say 'The way I could help you is . . .'"
- "Pick out some people here whom you would like to help with something they have shared, and try to greatly exaggerate a helpful attitude toward them."
- "If there is somebody in your life who has been a helper, see whether you can become that person, and go around to all members of the group and help them as that person would."

- "Pick out someone in the group who in some way reminds you of someone in your family whom you say you are tired of helping. Talk to that person about how it feels for you to help him or her and to get so little in return for yourself."

Why is Claude so anxious about letting others struggle on their own? Does he believe that the leader is not taking care of the group's needs and that he has to provide direction? These go-arounds give the leader a chance to discover Claude's motives. Perhaps he has believed all his life that no one will take care of him and that it is his duty to take care of everyone else. He may have been so burdened with taking responsibility for others that he does not see how he can behave any differently. To simply label him a Band-Aider is to ignore the dynamics his helpfulness may reveal. Eventually his work might be directed toward exploring ways in which he would like to be taken care of.

Why ask Claude to exaggerate being helpful when this is the behavior that seems to get in his way? By not trying to talk him out of how he feels, by giving him an opportunity to fully experience how he acts, the leader can get him to see clearly the implications of his behavior and to decide whether he wants to continue with his present style.

The leader could also use alternative strategies that involve cognitive restructuring in working with Claude:

- Ask Claude to list out loud all the reasons he has for helping others. Why is helping others so important? When did he make his decision that his place was to be so helpful?
- Ask the group to brainstorm on why Claude should be helpful, and then ask him to evaluate each of the comments. Here he may begin to challenge his assumption that he should be helpful.
- Suggest to Claude that he ask for something in return from each person he attempts to help. Here he has an opportunity to experiment with a dimension of his behavior that is undeveloped. This approach calls to his attention his giving style.
- Have group members say to Claude, each time he engages in helping behaviors, "You're helping me again, Claude!" This technique makes use of other members to monitor his behavior.
- Ask Claude to observe his behavior outside the group for a time and record instances in which he puts his own needs in second place. Through this self-monitoring process, he may see ways in which he resists receiving from others.

We want to make it clear that we are not against a helping attitude, nor would we want to try to get Claude to adopt a "me-first" attitude. Rather, the leader can use these techniques to help him discover for himself the one-sidedness of his interactions and how he affects others. His all-too-willing-to-help side can easily cause resentment in others, for they may feel continually indebted to him while at the same time having little to offer him. After he gets a clear picture of how his behavior affects others, he can decide whether he wants to change this aspect of his personality. The group provides the context for him to see himself as others perceive him, and then he is equipped to decide if and what he wants to change.

"Nobody ever listens to me." Julio says "Nobody ever listened to me when I was a kid, no one ever listened to me in school, no one ever listens to me at home, and I feel that no one listens to me here either." We might begin by asking Julio to pick out some members of the group who he feels are not listening to him and to say what leads him to believe that they aren't. Suppose he gets feedback from the group that suggests he is right—people have found themselves not paying much attention to him when he speaks. We might then try in several ways to discover what it is about him that causes people not to listen to him:

- Ask Julio if there is someone in the group whom he would especially like to have as a listener. He can then talk to that person.
- Ask Julio to become either of his parents and show how that parent might gain or lose the attention of the group members if that parent were in Julio's place.
- If Julio's voice is exceptionally flat and unmodulated, ask him to change the pitch of his voice.
- Explore what Julio might gain from not being heard by asking him to work with a sentence starting "If you really heard what I was saying, you would . . ."
- Ask some group members to give Julio specific feedback on the ways in which they perceive him as being difficult to listen to, and provide him with some suggestions that would increase his chances of being heard.
- Give him a homework assignment for the next week that will make explicit what we suspect are his underlying beliefs. Ask him to preface his remarks to people with "I know that what I am going to say isn't very worthwhile and you probably aren't going to listen to me, but . . ."

It might be a mistake to stay too concretely with Julio's first remarks. We want to be ready to pick up clues to what is really bothering him when he says he's not listened to. Maybe he has a history of feeling unloved and unimportant.

By using the techniques listed above, we are attempting to (1) get Julio to acknowledge his complaint and give him an opportunity to voice it, (2) get him to exaggerate those aspects of his behavior that might produce the situation of which he complains, (3) have others give feedback that will help him clarify what he might be doing or how others experience him, (4) have him discover where he might have learned to do what he does, (5) give him an opportunity to try out being different, and (6) give him feedback and, perhaps, positive reinforcement for what he chooses to do differently. These techniques are not aimed at changing Julio. They provide a context for him to discover what he does, where he learned it, how his behavior affects others, and how he could do things differently.

This example illustrates how to combine exploring the here and now with examining the client's past. Although work may often turn out to emphasize family dynamics during the client's childhood, we typically start the work by looking at present feelings within the group. Then, if past history becomes relevant, the group members have already been made to feel included in the struggle, and they are ready to stay with the individual's work on past history and share his excitement as they watch for a transformation in his present conduct.

"A part of me wants this, and a part of me wants that." Ambivalence, dichotomies, polarities—these are all extremely common in counseling work. Some common polarities are: "A part of me wants to stay with my family, but a part of me wants to go back to work." "A part of me wants to push you away, but a part of me wants to have you hold me." "A part of me loves my Dad, and a part of me hates him." "A part of me wants to live, but a part of me wants to die." "Sometimes I feel important; sometimes I feel worthless." "A part of me trusts you, and yet a part of me doesn't." "A part of me wants to feel; a part of me wants to go numb." Typically, we look for ways in which each part can be expressed and try to assure the client that each part will have a turn to be heard. In this way, the client need not constantly cancel the force of one side by considering the other side simultaneously.

Polarities can have different meanings. If Fred voices a polarity, are both parts really parts of him, or does he want one thing and introject the point of view of someone else who wants something different? If the two sides seem to genuinely represent him, our objective might be to seek a means of acknowledging both and integrating them. If he clearly wants one side but feels he is supposed to want the other side, our concern is to make this split clear and to present an opportunity to reject the foreign side.

One way to clarify the split is to accentuate it. A standard Gestalt technique is to ask Fred to sit in one chair while acting out one side and to sit in a different chair while being the other. This exercise has the advantage of bringing his whole body into play; movement symbolizes doing something rather than being stuck. And using two chairs allows us and Fred to clearly identify which side is being expressed. The moment he seems to be shifting to the other side in what he says, he should move to the other chair or be asked to do so.

We may look for clues about Fred's preference for one side or the other. Is his voice flat and dead in one chair, animated in the other? Is he comfortable in one chair, tense in the other? We are alert to the way he wants to go, and we follow his lead. Similarly, if he has introduced the dichotomy with "On the one hand . . . and on the other hand . . . ," we might ask him to let each of his hands represent a side. His clearly leaning to one side is a clue to his real preference.

In using a technique that accentuates polarities, the leader must be aware of when to request that Fred switch sides. The leader may not have to make the request; Fred may be aware of which side he is expressing and change chairs or hands accordingly. But he may need prompting to switch chairs if he unconsciously starts polluting one side with feelings from the other.

Polarities can also indicate that Fred is afraid to make a decision. In this case, however, he may prove to be much clearer about his choice than he wants to acknowledge. Sometimes all we have to say is "Pretend you do know which way to go," "Take a guess," or "What don't you want to know?"

Another approach might be to ask Fred to consciously stay with just one side of his dilemma for the next week and to allow it to become dominant. Or we might ask him to assume that one side wins out and that he must stay with that decision for the rest of his life. How would that feel?

The techniques mentioned so far do not include other group members in the work. As we have said many times before, we try to be constantly alert to the possibility of bringing in others who seem to be reacting or who have said something at another time that might connect with Fred's work. We also typically gear the exercises toward bringing in as many others as feasible, perhaps by using some of these techniques:

- Encourage others to share dichotomies of theirs that resemble Fred's.
- While Fred is speaking from one side, ask him to select someone else in the group to speak for the other side.
- Divide the group members according to which side of Fred's dilemma they feel closer to, and have a group dialogue.
- Ask Fred to sit in the middle of the group, and let others argue for the various sides.
- Have the group members vote on how they would prefer Fred to feel, and then ask him to persuade them to change their votes.

In this illustration with Fred and in several other cases we presented, the possibilities for involving other participants in one person's work have become evident.

"*I so much want your approval.*"   People often keep their thoughts to themselves out of fear that if they express themselves, they will not gain approval. They struggle with this issue in their everyday lives, and they also bring it to the group. Within a group, if there is a norm about being disclosing, these individuals experience a conflict between the pressure to participate and their desire to withhold for fear that others might not like what they say and do.

Herman asks for the leader's approval continually but indirectly. One technique here is for the leader to suggest that he tell her outright how desperately he wants her approval and that he write her every day of the following week discussing how much he desires this approval and describing all the things he has done that day that he hoped she would approve of. The rationale for using this technique is that by openly acknowledging what his behavior expresses, he may be able to see clearly what he is doing. Even if this exercise doesn't eliminate his need for approval, it allows him to control that need.

Another technique is to ask Herman "Is there anybody in the group from whom you particularly sense disapproval?" If he thinks that no one in the group disapproves of him, he can take on the role of each member of the group, pretend that the person disapproves, and say what disapproving thoughts he supposes that this person may have. The rationale for this technique is to uncover his projections. If he picks out someone in the group from whom he senses disapproval, the leader can ask him whom this person reminds him of and then have him speak to the imagined person.

Herman can then pretend that he is that disapproving member and, as such, can say something disapproving to each of the other members of the group. The rationale here is that along with his fear of being disapproved of, there might be a strong desire to be critical of others. He may find that his real fear is that others will be as critical as he is. Often those who have an excessive need for approval are also critical. An expected outcome is that this technique will both open up the group and bring Herman's own repressed hostility into the open.

When a client like Herman is trying out a different side to his personality—for example, acknowledging a disapproving side—it helps to connect this work with a different posture. While he is speaking critically to others in the group, he is sitting on the floor with his arms hugging his knees. The leader might say "Herman, as you continue with this exercise, I'd like for you to stand up straight and point to each person as you say something disapproving to him or her." One outcome may be that he will discover that his suppressed criticalness can be constructive and that, besides, he becomes a more interesting person when he lets this side of him show.

"I'm empty inside." Adeline says she is afraid to work anymore: "My greatest fear is that if I do look at myself, I'll find that I'm empty and am simply a reflection of what everyone else expects. Now, at least, I can kid myself by saying that maybe I'm not so bad after all; yet if I really looked, I just might find nothing inside. Maybe I don't have anything to offer anyone." In this case, Adeline may really feel empty inside or fear that she is empty, but she may also be holding back material that she is afraid to acknowledge to herself or the group. In developing a technique for working with her, the leader needs to be prepared to pursue either direction.

A common mistake of beginning group leaders, and group members as well, in a case like this one is to try to talk Adeline out of what she says she is feeling, to assure her that she does have a great deal going on inside her. Instead, the leader might encourage her to experience even more fully what she feels.

Another common mistake is for the leader to assume too quickly that he knows what Adeline's words mean, rather than allowing her to say what being empty means to her. The leader can ask her to select a visual image that symbolizes being empty. Suppose she picks a dead tree stump that is hollow inside. The leader can then direct her to become the hollow stump. She may say: "I'm dead and useless. I'm rotten and decaying inside, of no use or value. There's no life left in me, nothing but dead and useless wood." Now the leader can try to have Adeline move from symbolic to concrete language, taking his clues from words she uses that seem to invoke the most feeling in her and from whatever he happens to know already about her: "You mentioned being useless. Would you talk more about ways in which you're feeling useless in your life?" Or: "You describe yourself as rotten inside. I wonder what's so rotten in there." These promptings may be sufficient to involve her on a feeling level in pursuing these themes. If she does not yet get close to much feeling, the leader can ask her to tell other members something about herself that is rotten, decaying, dead, or empty.

Or if the leader suspects that what Adeline is saying connects significantly with the concerns of another member of the group, he can ask her to talk to this member about her emptiness. Another possibility is to ask her to talk to a member of the group whom she experiences as being full of life. By doing this exercise, she may discover that she hides behind her sense of deadness because she is jealous of those who seem more alive.

Although people who say they have nothing to offer others often lack confidence, there could be a hidden arrogance in their remark. They may feel that others have nothing to offer them. To explore this possibility with Adeline, the leader might ask her to tell group members something about them that she suspects is dead or hollow.

During the course of these exercises, Adeline may reveal that her sense of emptiness comes from the fact that she has devoted years to raising a family. Now that her children have lives of their own, she no longer feels she has anything to offer. In contrast, she experiences others in the group as still young and vital and moving forward in their lives. Thus, the technique will have brought material into the open in a way that promotes spontaneous interaction among the members of the group.

As an extension of her work, Adeline might take home a piece of dead wood as a reminder of what she explored and be asked to write each day for half an hour about all the ways in which she feels empty. She can bring her journal to the next meeting of the group and tell the members how it felt to allow herself to be empty and dead for part of each day. The rationale again is to give her an opportunity to fully experience her sense of emptiness, because once she stops running away from her fear that she is empty, she is more able to determine how much truth there is in it. If she does discover some aspects of her life that are without meaning, she is then in a position to change her life in ways that could result in a fuller sense of purpose.

Another way of working with Adeline is through the use of a guided fantasy. The advantage of this technique is that it includes the entire group. These might be the instructions: "I'd like to explore this feeling with you by starting out with a guided fantasy. The rest of you in the group might try going along with it to see what it brings up for you. Imagine some scene that represents emptiness to you. It might be a barren landscape, a dark empty house, or whatever you like. Now I want to ask you to imagine entering this empty place—trying to be there. Let yourself feel the emptiness of the place you have entered. As you do so, tell yourself that what you are really doing is entering yourself and that you find that there is nothing there. Now I'd like for you to talk about what you notice as missing. For example, if you find yourself thinking that there is no capacity for feeling or for loving within this empty place, talk about that. I'd like to know more about what you call your emptiness."

Depending on where this technique goes, the leader can then perhaps try this exercise: "Now I would like to ask you to look around the room at the others, and when you see someone who you think has some quality that you find yourself empty of, tell that person about it. If you would like to take some of that quality from that person to fill your emptiness, tell what it would be like to have that quality." This technique gives Adeline an opportunity to be specific about what she means by being empty inside and also promotes working with others in the group.

In this example, the techniques are designed primarily to provide Adeline with an opportunity to experience her emptiness as fully as possible as well as to acquire some insight into what she does that contributes to her feeling of being empty. If the leader believes that action on Adeline's part is also essential if she expects to change, he can challenge her to think of concrete steps she can begin to take to deal with her emptiness in a constructive way. Eventually, Adeline may devise a plan involving new behavior designed to bring some meaning to her life. For example, she may decide to do some things that she has been saying she wants to do but has never found the time to do.

"People just don't appreciate me." Bonnie wants to work on her feeling that people do not recognize her or appreciate her. She says: "No matter what I do or how hard I try, I still feel unappreciated. My kids are demanding, and I feel they just use me. What's more, my husband rarely gives me support or tells me that I mean anything to him. He is demanding too, and I'm left feeling that I'm never enough. Even in this group I often feel unrecognized. I feel that I don't count and that what I do in here—or what I am—is not appreciated."

We might ask Bonnie to identify and talk to those members of the group (including the leaders) by whom she feels least appreciated. While she is doing this exercise, we pay attention to her style. Is she especially timid or affectless? Is there anything else about her that invites people not to take her seriously? We also want to find out specifically what she means by appreciation and get information about what she may want. We might give her an opportunity to list all the things for which she is not receiving appreciation.

If we suspect from what she says that her feeling of not being appreciated has been with her from childhood, we might ask her to relive a scene with her parents when she felt unappreciated. She can be herself as a child and talk to her mother and father, using substitutes selected from the group, about what she is feeling: "Go back to that time, be that child, and, as if your parents were here now, say some of the things that you might have wanted to say to them." Bonnie may say: "You don't recognize me for what I do. Nothing I do is good enough for you."

Then we might ask Bonnie to become either of her parents, with someone else in the group playing the part of Bonnie. Bonnie, as one of her parents, can talk about how nothing Bonnie does is good enough. She can imitate a parent's style of talking with her and attempt to express some of the things she fantasizes that her parents may have left unsaid. By having Bonnie's substitute enter into this dialogue, we can involve another person in her work and also give her an opportunity to see how she comes across. The substitute may also give her some ideas for an alternative and potentially more forceful style. This technique encourages her to verbalize some of the feelings she had as a child and then perhaps to discover how she may presently be encouraging people to treat her in the way she felt treated then.

These techniques can be followed with various cognitive approaches aimed at challenging the beliefs that influence Bonnie's behavior. In a number of ways she can be urged to critically evaluate her assumption that regardless of what she accomplishes, it will never be enough. Some directions for further work can be found in these open-ended questions:

- "What will you have to do to feel that you *are* enough? Who is the person from whom you are seeking this external confirmation, and, even if you attain this validation, will you *then* be enough?"
- "How are you contributing to your feelings of inadequacy by clinging to the assumption that others *must* appreciate you?"
- "How valid is your conviction that you don't count unless others appreciate you?"

In general, the goal is to provide a context for Bonnie to think critically about how her assumptions and beliefs determine how she feels. She is likely to feel and behave differently if she successfully challenges some of her self-defeating beliefs.

"I don't like being overweight." Frances is concerned about being overweight, but at the same time she says she likes who she is and is angry that people consider her heavy: "After all, 50 pounds overweight is not that bad." In this case, the leader needs to attend to the mixed message that Frances is sending. She says simultaneously that she does not like being overweight and that "50 pounds is not that bad." One approach is to ask Frances "If 50 pounds is not that bad, why are you bringing up this issue?" She can be helped to decide what she would like to do with her statement. Does she want to deal with being 50 pounds overweight, or does she want to deal with people who perceive her as being heavy? Might she want to explore both issues?

Assume that Frances would like to deal with both her own concerns about being overweight and people who think she is too heavy. The leader could suggest that she do a go-around and tell each member something that she would like to say to those who tell her that she is too heavy. Once she completes this exercise, there will probably be a number of clues that point the way to another technique aimed at further exploration of how she is affected by those who see her as being overweight.

If Frances is still willing to pursue *her* concerns about her weight, it is possible to create an exercise that will assist her in sorting out her feelings and how they affect her self-esteem. The leader can ask her to pick up some heavy object and continue to talk about whether she ought to try losing weight. When asked to stand before another member to tell him or her how it is to hold this object, she says: "I can't. I can't move over there easily enough. I'm too inhibited by carrying this heavy thing around."

Eventually, Frances may pause and reflect on the symbolic significance of the exercise and of her words. The leader can then ask her to repeat some of what she has said, replacing references to the heavy object with references to her own body weight. By speaking symbolically and then concretely, she may be able to reveal the limitations she feels herself to have as a result of her weight. When she finally drops the burden she is carrying around, she may remark: "I feel so light and free. I never knew how heavy 50 pounds could be. I've become so used to them I had no idea how much of a strain these extra pounds are." The group may comment on the way she held onto the object even though the leader had not instructed her to continue holding this object.

At the end of the session Frances may declare her intention to go to a gym, which she was previously embarrassed to do. The leader can ask her to do a homework assignment when in the gym: occasionally pick up 50 pounds and reflect on what she has learned during her work in the group.

In this example, the resistance Frances probably would have felt to acknowledging that her extra weight was cumbersome and prevented her from getting close to people was bypassed by being approached symbolically. No one pushed her into losing weight; she had an opportunity to acknowledge her own dissatisfaction with those 50 pounds. It needs to be emphasized that a good deal of trust on the part of Frances, as well as a high level of trust within the group, are required for this exercise to be effectively and sensitively used.

In our work with members who bring up concerns about being overweight and how it affects their self-image, we typically find that the weight is only symptomatic of a deeper concern. We often tend to focus on the deeper struggle, and interestingly, people frequently lose weight when they begin to appreciate themselves for the persons they are. Sometimes they are harshly critical of themselves if they judge themselves to be in noncomformity with a societal standard of having an ideal body. If they are able to ease up on their self-critical attitudes and decide for themselves that they want to lose weight, they are more likely to experience success than if they persist with weight-control plans because of someone besides themselves.

In this example, we described how props can be used productively to intensify work. Even though what follows is not directly related to being overweight, we list some other possibilities for using props to sharpen a point and to help members explore an area that concerns them:

- Ask a member to hide behind a blanket as she talks about her desire to hide.
- Surround a member with cushions and pillows to emphasize his fear of getting close and his desire for distance.
- Have a member who feels that she has little time for anything hold a clock or an egg timer.
- Ask participants to collect items that have some personal meaning for them: a rock, a branch, a leaf, an empty beer can, a book, a key, some fruit, a cigarette. The object can serve as a reminder for some action.
- Have a member hold a small pillow and talk to it as a child.
- Have a member use a stack of cushions to represent people who are the targets of her anger.
- Have a member use an art object to stimulate fantasy.
- Have a member who wants to unload guilt put these feelings in a can (or bucket, box, wastebasket) and give them to the leader to keep.
- Have a member who would like to leave behind some painful experience go over to the cabinet and "file" this particular memory.

With some of these props, there is value in allowing members to act as if they were free of some burden, at least for a while. For instance, if Cynthia puts her guilt over an affair into a container, she can begin a process of releasing her guilt. The leader could say: "I'll keep your guilt in this container, so you won't have to worry about it for this week. If you want your guilt back next week, then we can talk about it, and it will still be in this container if you decide to reclaim it." The seriousness of a member's words should not be sidestepped, for they will provide rich clues for pursuing the direction the work takes. These techniques cannot undo intense feelings such as guilt, shame, rage, and abandonment. Such techniques are not meant to solve problems but to help a participant consider for a time what her life might be like without the guilt or hurt that she has been carrying for years. All props, of course, are designed for intensifying a member's work, not to entertain the group. At times the participants might be entertained, but this should never be done at a member's expense, nor is this the basic purpose of using props in techniques.

"What I got out of that is . . ." Often people quickly forget some of the most significant insights or lessons that emerge in work they do in a group. Some therapists believe that people remember what they are ready to remember, but we disagree. We think that even though catharsis and insight are not followed by a lasting decision to change, clients can profit by thinking about what they want to be able to recall later on. Tim's emotions are now subsiding, but he has just been through 20 minutes of work on several themes. He began by discussing a conflict he had been having with another member. In the feedback exercise that followed, other members praised him for several of his traits but criticized him for his sarcasm. This feedback led to role playing in which he imitated some of the sarcasm he recalled his mother directing at his father. He then began sobbing over the death of his father, and this work triggered grieving in several members of the group. Now, as things are calming down, we ask Tim what he wants to learn from this work. Somewhat to our disappointment he replies "What I got out of that is that I'm as sarcastic as my mother was and that people don't like me for it." We had hoped he would remember more than just negative feedback, although remembering only negative generalities is a frequent outcome of work in groups. What can we do? Here are some possible techniques we could introduce at this point:

- Ask Tim to review each phase of the work he has just done and summarize the specifics.
- Invite members to tell Tim what they most hope he will remember.
- Ask Tim to take on the role of each person who gave him feedback and repeat, as best he can, what that person said.
- Ask every member who is willing to do so to write in Tim's journal something that he or she wants Tim to remember.
- Ask Tim to describe how he might discount what he got from his work.
- Ask Tim to go around the group explaining to each person who gave him feedback how he might discount that feedback or put it in the most negative light. (For example, he might say he thought June was merely flattering him when she said she found him attractive.)
- Give Tim the homework assignment of writing in his journal about what happened in his work.
- Ask Tim to look around the room and impress on his memory the faces of the members of the group as they look right now after having just been so intensely involved in his work. Ask him to try to recall the way these people look when, in weeks to come, he thinks back on today's work.
- Ask Tim to pretend that his mother and his father are in the room and to role-play each of them in summarizing what has been said.
- Ask Tim to name three or four specific lessons he wants to remember from what he has just experienced and to stand up as he declares these lessons to the group.

In the next chapter we discuss techniques for consolidating lessons learned from a group session and for remembering lessons learned over the whole life of a group. We want to emphasize here that the process of reviewing and consolidating insights and formulating decisions about what to put into practice in daily life should be continually encouraged. The completion of a highly emotional segment of a session is a particularly appropriate time to create and introduce techniques highlighting lessons to be learned.

Concluding Comments

In this chapter we have addressed the common themes that a group typically explores during the working stage. Our aim is to create and use techniques to facilitate the exploration of material that emerges from the interactions within the group. It is important to take our clues from our clients and then devise techniques that will help them understand how they are thinking, feeling, and behaving. We tend to avoid using planned techniques or structured exercises as catalysts. We hope that we have made the point that techniques are most powerful when they are designed for a specific situation in a group as well as for the personality and therapeutic style of the leader. There is no "right" way to proceed with the material that members produce. Instead, there are many ways of creatively working with members to help them gain self-awareness and to provide them with the encouragement to make changes they most want to make. It is essential that you think about the rationale for the techniques you use and that you be able to discuss what you hope to accomplish by using them. Finally, at all times techniques must be used with respect and concern for the client. They are merely tools to facilitate self-understanding, not ends in themselves.

Questions and Activities

1. Review our account of the characteristics of the working stage of a group. Think about a group that you have led or in which you have been a member, and describe how it did or did not attain this stage. Think about a group that you have been in that did not reach the working stage, and evaluate why it did not do so.
2. A member of your group says "Last week I felt very close to people in the group, and this week I'm feeling as if I want to withdraw." How would you handle this remark? What might you say? Would what occurred the prior week be something that you'd want to address?
3. Dee says that she can't talk to her parents. Develop several different hunches about what might be involved in this issue for her, and explain different ways in which you might want to work with her.
4. Someone says "I'm afraid to look at what I'm really like inside." You suggest that she stand inside a closet and talk to the group about what she is feeling. The client declares an unwillingness to follow your suggestion and is clearly anxious about the idea. What might you do now?
5. Assuming that transferences typically occur in most groups, how would you utilize this phenomenon for furthering group work? What kinds of questions could you ask of a member that might elicit the admission of the transference? One such question is "Who in the group could be your father?"
6. In asking Carlos to speak in his native language, the leader assumed that his feelings would be intensified by speaking as he might have spoken when the issues he was working on were more pressing. Explain some of your views about the possible connection between how one talks and one's intensity of feeling, and describe some techniques that you think might amplify this connection. What advantages, if any, do you see to asking a person like Carlos to speak in his native language? How might

you make use of others in the group who share his native tongue? How might you bring into this work others in the room who do not speak that language?

7. After reviewing our suggestions for working with Judy's remark that she feels the burdens of the world, read a discussion of the dynamics of depression in a textbook on abnormal psychology, and develop some alternative techniques for working with her statement.

8. Imagine a specific population you might work with, and suppose that a member of such a group were to ask you: "Why do we have to share our feelings? What good does that do?" What would you say? How would your response depend on the population? Would it depend on the stage of the group?

9. In discussing Claude's wanting to be helpful, we proposed that his attitude might have an inhibiting effect on others in the group. Develop a technique designed to explore how others in the group are affected by his style. If you were to ask him to exaggerate being helpful, what would your theoretical rationale be? What might be the effect of asking him to do an exercise in which he avoids being helpful?

10. People have different ways of expressing their feelings and thoughts, and their styles may work well for them. However, they may be subjected to group pressure to express themselves in other ways. What are your thoughts on this pressure, and what are some responses you might make if you were to observe group pressure to conform to a norm?

11. In the example of Julio, who feels that no one listens to him, we talk about the relevance of past history. If you are using this book as part of a class, have the class divide for a debate on the pros and cons of working on past material in a group. Do you think that a behavioral viewpoint excludes considering an individual's past? What about a Gestalt or an existential point of view?

12. Betty says she is confused. In the example, the leader used a technique for joining her in her resistance. If you used this technique, how would you explain to a colleague or fellow student your rationale? Invent some techniques for directly confronting the resistance, and compare these with the approach we suggest.

13. Do some reading on Carl Jung and on Fritz Perls. How would you incorporate what they say about polarities into techniques you might invent for working with Fred and his ambivalence?

14. Suppose a member of your group says that you are not sharing enough of yourself. How would you handle this remark if it was made during the working stage of a group? What factors would you take into consideration? To what extent do you see your style as self-disclosing or as stating your own feelings or experiences?

15. In discussing Adeline's feeling of being empty inside, we suggested a guided-fantasy exercise. Write a guided fantasy you might use, and explain what you would expect to accomplish with the imagery you employ.

16. Develop a homework assignment for Adeline designed to have her explore her sense of emptiness in everyday life. Develop a different assignment designed to help her challenge any irrational beliefs she may have about her emptiness.

17. Bonnie says that people don't appreciate her. Describe a context in which you might ask the group to sing to her "My Bonnie Lies over the Ocean." When and why might you ask Bonnie to sing this song? What might you hope to accomplish, and how might the result you hope for come about? When might you ask her to make up her own song about people not appreciating her, and why might you ask her to do so?

18. Adlerians believe that our overall goals are fictional ideals we cannot test in reality and that our lives are based on such fictions. What might be the fictional ideal implicit in Bonnie's remark about people not appreciating her, and how might you develop a technique to explore this fictional ideal?

19. During the working stage it is still important to continue to ask members to engage in evaluating their progress in the group to determine the degree to which they are attaining their objectives. What are some ways in which you would help members assess the degree of satisfaction with their participation at this stage?

20. We describe Carl as being afraid to get close to people because of childhood injunctions (parental messages). What are some injunctions you received as a child? Are any of your injunctions similar to those of Carl? If so, if you were to self-disclose to him, what might you say? Devise some contracts and homework assignments that you think might encourage him to challenge his injunctions.

21. Assume that Frances is serious about wanting to lose weight. Do some reading on behavioral approaches to losing weight, and set up a behavioral plan for her. Include devising specific goals, monitoring behavior, and developing reinforcements. How would you assess the effectiveness of your plan?

22. Cheryl says that the real world is not like the group. If you were her group leader and wanted to explain your views on this issue, what would you say? What techniques might be appropriate for bridging gaps between what group and real life are like?

23. Jane shows a reluctance to cry. Do you think it important for her to cry? Explain.

24. We are more concerned with what people do not say with respect to fears and feelings than with what they do say in a group. What is your view on this topic?

25. What role would the cultural backgrounds of the participants in your group play in deciding which kinds of techniques to use or not to use? Do you have any guidelines for how you might modify certain techniques to fit a group that is made up of culturally diverse clients?

26. Suppose that you are leading by yourself a group in which several people are simultaneously expressing intense emotion. How might you react

to this situation? What might you do if you were frightened by the intensity of their emotions? How would you most like to be as a leader in this context? Describe a situation in which this phenomenon develops, and describe some techniques you might employ.

27. Do you see any exploration of dreams as valuable in group work? What reservations, if any, do you have about working with an individual's dream in a group? What techniques would maximize the opportunity for others in the group to be involved in working on one person's dream?

28. How might Melissa's dream about the group be a manifestation of transference, and what techniques might you introduce to explore this possibility?

29. Do some reading on the Gestalt approach to working with dreams. How might you work with Patty's dream and with Melissa's dream using Gestalt methods?

30. What value might there be in asking members to simply share their dreams without attempting to interpret them? What impact might this technique have on group cohesion?

31. What kinds of mistakes might you fear making as a group leader? How might your fear get in the way of your trying new techniques? How might you react to mistakes you make in a group?

32. Your group members believe that a technique you suggested for one of them was a mistake, but you think your suggestion was appropriate. What would you do?

33. We encourage members to gain some cognitive grasp of material they have expressed on an emotional level. We hold that much will be lost if members are not encouraged to think about their work in a group. Many counselors would not agree that putting things into a cognitive framework and attempting to summarize lessons are important. What is your view, and why?

34. Our position is that if you have prepared your group during the initial stage, the group will largely take care of itself during the working stage. Do you agree? Why or why not?

35. For yourself, what importance do you place on having experienced as a group member any of the techniques that you are likely to introduce in a group that you are leading? To what degree do you think your own experiences as a client in a group can enable you to effectively facilitate a group for others? What are some specific ways in which you can use your membership experience to help members work in depth on their issues?

CHAPTER SEVEN

Techniques for the Final Stage

Techniques for Ending a Session

Techniques for Terminating a Group

Techniques for Continuing Assessment and Follow Up

Techniques for Evaluating a Group

Concluding Comments

Questions and Activities

In this chapter we discuss termination of individual sessions and of the life of the group, an often-neglected topic. Many leaders simply and abruptly announce that a group is at an end. They make no attempt to integrate, or bring together, lessons that could be learned from the group experience. Because such learning does not happen automatically, it should be fostered and structured throughout the entire life of a group. Perhaps the two most important phases of a group are its beginning and its end—the beginning, because that is where the tone of the group is set; the end, because that is where learning is consolidated and action plans are typically formulated. We need to stress again that in an effectively functioning group, the members are striving to carry what they are learning in the sessions into their everyday lives. They do this by formulating plans to carry out between the sessions, by making a commitment to do homework assignments, and by practicing a variety of new behaviors outside of the group. Leaders need to pay attention to the endings of every session, and they also need to teach members how to apply the skills they are acquiring to coping with the challenges facing them at home, work, and school. Yet some specific tasks demand attention as the group approaches its conclusion.

Avoiding acknowledging a group's completion may reflect an unconscious desire on the part of the leader or members not to deal with the role that endings play in their lives. When termination is not dealt with, the group misses an opportunity to explore an area about which many members have profound feelings. Even more important, much of what clients take away from a group is likely to be lost and forgotten if they do not make a sustained effort to review and think through the specifics of work they have done.

In general, the following tasks need to be accomplished during the final stage of the group:

- Members can be encouraged to face the inevitable ending of the group and to discuss fully their feelings of separation.
- Members can complete any unfinished business they have with other members or the leaders.
- Members can be taught how to leave the group and how to carry with them what they have learned.
- Members can be assisted in making specific plans for change and in taking concrete steps to put the lessons they have learned into effect in their daily lives.
- Leaders can help members discover ways of creating their own support systems after they leave the group.
- Specific plans for follow-up work and evaluation can be made.

Techniques for Ending a Session

Throughout the life of a group, the leader should remain aware of time and should teach the participants how best to use the limited time available to them. One of the pitfalls for inexperienced therapists is being unaware of how much time is left in a session. Such leaders may open up material when it would be more valuable to start consolidating what has been accomplished. Their behavior reinforces the tendency of group members to bring up new material at the last minute (a form of resistance), and it encourages members to manipulate the leaders into extending the session. It can also lead members to believe that leaders are inadequate or insensitive. For instance, Joan may typically bring up burning issues at the end of the session and then leave complaining of feeling cut off and ignored or of being left hanging. In the early stages of a group these complaints can set the stage for distrust or dissatisfaction.

Asking members to sum up. A good practice is to allow at least ten minutes at the end of a session, depending on the length of the session and the size of the group, for members to summarize what the session has meant to them individually. These are some of the questions they can be asked to answer:

- "Could you briefly summarize what this session has meant to you?"
- "What steps are you willing to take between now and our next session toward making changes in your life?"
- "Was there anything unfinished for you today that you would like to continue in our next meeting?"
- "What was the most important thing you experienced during this meeting?"
- "Could you summarize the important thoughts or insights you're taking with you?"
- "What touched you most in other people's work today?"
- "Before we go, is there any feedback you want to give to someone else here?"
- "What did you learn about yourself?"
- "Is there anything you want to be committed to doing between now and the next time we meet?"
- "Is there anything you regret not working on during this session that you would like to at least mention before we close?"
- "Did you get what you wanted from this session?"
- "Are you satisfied with your level of participation in this session?"
- "If you are apathetic, bored, uninvolved, hostile, or resistant, what are you willing to do (if anything) to change this attitude?"

This practice of making at least a quick check of every member is extremely important, for it challenges members each week to think about what they are both giving to and getting from the group. If they report that they are pleased with what they are experiencing, they can be asked to be specific about what they like and to describe anything they'd like to see more of. If they report that they are not pleased (with the group itself, the leader, or themselves), they can be encouraged to be specific both about what they'd want changed and about their plans for making these changes either in the group or in themselves. If this check is made regularly, members are less likely to complain at the termination of the group that they got nothing from it and that no attempt was made to improve work in the group.

Dealing with unfinished work.   What if intense work in a session is not going to be finished by the time the group ends? First, there is nothing inherently terrible or catastrophic about members leaving the group with their emotions stirred up, although it is important for them to verbalize how they are feeling. The sensitive leader can help bring a sense of closure simply by acknowledging those feelings that are left hanging. Second, clients often accomplish more than one might suppose in a fairly short period, especially if the leader has let the time constraints be known. People automatically pace their work to the time they know they have.

The leader may tone things down and still give the client something constructive to work with by saying: "I know that a lot has been stirred up in you that we're not going to have time to really work through today. But before we leave, I'd like each of you to say a sentence or two about what you're leaving with today and where you'd like to take this work during the week and in a future session." Another related approach at this point is simply to ask the client "Since we're running out of time for exploring this today, would you be willing to try to reflect on it a bit between now and the next meeting and bring it up again then?"

What do you do if a member moves into a deeply emotional issue as the minutes for a session are running out? Generally, members will pace themselves fairly well if the leaders remind them occasionally of how much time remains, particularly if the group norm is to keep within the scheduled boundaries. With the member who habitually brings up dramatic material that is likely to be left hanging, this pattern needs to be explored. But in spite of one's best efforts, there will be occasions when something will start to develop near the end of a session that will pose a dilemma of either giving up the time structure or seeming to be insensitive. These scenarios can often be spotted as they start to develop, and the leader can defuse the situation somewhat by a comment that makes the problem explicit. For instance: "John, it seems to me you're getting into some things that we're not going to have time to really explore today. Since we're going to have to stop pretty soon, I wonder if you'd be able to stand back a bit from the feelings that seem to be coming up, and just list and summarize the key things that we can try to come back to at the next meeting." Here the leader's phrasing is intended to convey empathy for John's predicament in being left with the issues coming up; the situation is salvaged about as well as one could hope if the issues are identified and acknowledged and John is helped to cast things into a form that won't leave him too "raw."

Some leaders make the mistake of thinking that unless a concern is brought to a finish, that issue is lost forever. This is rarely the case. If the issue is an important one, it can easily be returned to, especially if the member makes a commitment to bring it up at the next session, when there will be sufficient time to explore it. A leader can remind the client of this commitment at the following meeting by saying: "John, I remember that during the last session you experienced a lot of intensity related to an issue with your father. I wonder whether you had any more feelings about that or if there is anything you might want to say now to continue with that." Often the client will say: "I don't feel that anymore. That's no longer present for me." However, if John is willing to try to talk for a moment about what he was experiencing during the previous session, without worrying about whether it seems especially here and now, he may well be able to get into those feelings again.

In a sense, something is always going on at the end of every session. What matters is that whatever is going on be identified and summarized as much as possible. It is unrealistic to think that all members will bring to closure the issues they have raised in a meeting, and it is a mistake to attempt premature closure on an issue. Leaders should be careful to avoid "fixing up" a member's problem largely because of the need to see that everyone leaves feeling satisfied. It is often constructive for clients to leave with a sense of incompleteness, something to think about after the session and work with in future sessions. If people leave feeling too comfortable, they may not be motivated to reflect on what occurred in the session.

Arranging homework assignments.   One technique for closing a session and linking it to the next is to have members announce homework assignments or some means of carrying further the work they have done in a session and then to report on these assignments at the beginning of the next session. Homework can be devised by the members themselves, by the leader, or by other members of the group. Too often members do little thinking about or working on a personal issue they explored during a session, unless they commit themselves to doing so. For example, if Maria is fearful of dealing with her professors, she can commit herself to seeking out a professor before the next session and talking with the professor about her fears in the class. If she takes the ultimate responsibility for deciding on the nature of her assignment, she is already taking steps toward change.

Making your own comments and polling members.   Leaders can make a practice of giving their reactions, a group-process commentary, and a summary of the meeting toward the end of the session. Leaders might comment on the cohesion of the group, the degree to which members freely brought up topics for work, their willingness to take risks and talk about unsafe topics, the degree to which they interacted with one another (as opposed to speaking only directly to and through the leader), and their willingness to discuss negative concerns or feelings. Leaders might also write notes about each session during the week and then use these comments at the beginning of the next session as a catalyst for linking sessions. Members can also write down at the end of each session specific topics, questions, concerns, problems, or personal issues that they'd be willing to talk about in the next session. They are thus encouraged to think before the next session about what they've committed themselves to bring up. Although some therapists may think that this practice is too forced or planned, it is one technique for confronting members with their responsibility to use the limited time available to them in a group to its fullest. Another way to close each session is to set aside the last five minutes for members to fill out a brief assessment or rating sheet. These assessments give the leaders a continuing sense of how members are perceiving the group. The rating sheets can be tallied up in a few minutes, and the results can be presented at the beginning of the next session, especially if trends are noted. A rating scale from 1 to 10 can be used. Members can rate themselves, other members, and the leaders on some of the following dimensions (the leaders might fill out these forms too):

- To what degree were you involved in this session?
- To what degree did you want to be in the group today?
- To what degree did you see yourself as an active, contributing member of the group today?
- To what degree were you willing to take risks in the group?
- To what degree did you trust other members in the group today?
- To what degree did you trust the group leader today?
- To what degree has today's session stimulated you to think about your problems, your life situation, or possible decisions you might want to make?
- To what degree did today's group touch you emotionally or help you recall emotionally laden events in your life?
- To what degree did you care about other members in this session?
- To what degree were you willing to share what you were feeling and thinking in the session today?
- To what degree did you have clear goals for this session?
- To what degree are you willing to actively practice some new behavior this week?
- At this point, to what degree are you eager to return to the group next week?
- To what degree did you prepare yourself or think about this session before you came today?
- To what degree do you see the group as being alive, goal-directed, and energetic?
- To what degree do you think the group is cohesive and together at this time?
- To what degree are you willing to give others in the group feedback?
- To what degree are you willing to nondefensively take in the feedback you receive and consider it carefully?
- To what degree do you see this group as a positive force in helping you make the changes in your life that you want to make?
- To what degree did you see the group as productive today?

If the leaders tally up the results and see clear trends such as a lack of involvement, a low level of risk taking, an absence of trust, a limited amount of sharing, resistance to returning to the group, and an absence of cohesion, they can open the next session with a remark such as this one: "For the past two weeks most of you have apparently seen this group as a place where you don't feel safe to reveal personal material. Many of you agree that caring is absent, that goals are unclear, and that the energy level of the group is low. I'd like to have us look at this trend and see what we want to do about this situation, especially since we have a number of group sessions left." The members can then bring out some of their perceptions and openly evaluate the group, and the members and leaders can make decisions about changing the group's direction.

In summary, if leaders lose sight of the approaching end of a session, they have no choice but to announce abruptly "Well, group, we've run out of time; see you next week." If this practice becomes the norm, there is no closure for a session, no evaluation of accountability, and no concrete planning for the upcoming session.

Techniques for Terminating a Group

It is both ethically and clinically good practice to promote the termination of members from the group in the most efficient period of time. To accomplish this aim, group counselors monitor the progress made by each member and periodically invite the members to explore and reevaluate their experiences in the group.

Preparing for termination. In open groups, or those with changing membership, the matter of termination may need to be addressed each week. If Sarah will be leaving the group, her departure needs to be announced ahead of time so that she can deal with her feelings about leaving this group. Also, others in the group will probably have things to say to her about her leaving.

In closed groups with a fixed life span, the issue of termination must be faced well before the last session. Group members should be encouraged to express their feelings about the group's ending and to identify what more they want to do before the opportunity is gone. If the group is cohesive, members also need to deal with the sense of loss they may feel when the group is over.

When the end of the group is still a fair time away, the fact that an end will come can be used to motivate people to work. In the case of a time-limited group, the leaders can point out that the time is passing and that the group will eventually be ending. It is a good practice for leaders to stress the urgency of making full use of the limited time a group has and to help members assess how well they are making use of this time. Members cannot assume that they have plenty of time for getting around to their work. If they do, they will probably feel a sense of dissatisfaction when the final meeting arrives. Some members say: "It took me a long time to know what I wanted and to feel trusting in here. Now that this group is almost over, I feel I could begin to do some real work."

Leaders can use questions such as the following ones to prompt members to work: "Assume that this is the last chance you're going to have in this group to explore what you want. How do you want to use this time?" "If this were the last session of this group, how would you feel about what you've done, and what would you wish you had done differently?"

In addition, as the end of the group approaches, and preferably not at the last meeting, members can explore feelings they may have about the ending of the group and parallels with separation and death in their lives. Leaders should not underestimate the likelihood that the group has become for several of the participants a powerful family symbol or a focus of hope and of the possibility for change. They should have ample opportunity to explore these associations.

Leaders should also be alert to signs that the members are avoiding dealing with the group's ending. When members start introducing topics that they worked on long before, when the work in the group seems lacking in intensity, when there is much lateness, joking, or intellectualizing, members may be signaling through such resistance their unwillingness to leave. The leaders' own willingness to initiate the topic of termination can be excellent modeling here.

Reviewing highlights of the group experience.   Much of what members learn in a group will be lost unless certain devices are used to help them recall these lessons and to apply what they've learned in their everyday lives. One such device is to ask members to spontaneously recall moments they shared together: "I'd like each of you to close your eyes and imagine all the events during the time we've been together. Let yourself imagine that you have these events on videotape, that you can play back these tapes and actually see and remember what occurred in the group. Now let yourself go back to our very first session, and for a few minutes just sit with your eyes closed and see whatever comes to you about this first session. What do you remember feeling? How did people look to you then?" After a couple of minutes the leader can ask members to share freely and randomly glimpses of what they remember of this early session. Then the leader can say: "Now close your eyes again, and for a few minutes sit in silence and just let this tape go through your mind. Let whatever comes to mind get sharper and more focused. Remember whatever stands out for you. What were some of the events that you recall most clearly and that had the most meaning for you? Whenever you feel ready, just let yourself speak and share with the rest of us what you're remembering."

This technique of recalling special moments may bring back to life incidents of conflict in the group, of closeness and warmth, of humor and lightness, of pain, or of tension and anxiety. The more members can verbalize their experiences and the more they can recall what actually happened in the group, the greater their chances of integrating and using the lessons they have learned.

Fred, for example, says: "I'm thinking about the time when the members in here told me that although I appeared tough, they saw a tender side of me deep down. That helped me a great deal to feel that it was acceptable to *have feelings*, although I must admit that I still have a long way to go before I feel OK about expressing these feelings openly." Sue mentions the time that she confronted the group leader and relates: "I can still feel myself shaking as I let myself get angry at you. That was a new feeling for me to feel *and* express my anger to authority figures, and I learned that the world doesn't fall apart when I do get angry." Barbara recalls: "In one session there was this heavy silence in the room, which felt terribly uncomfortable to me. I wanted to say something to break the tension in the room. It was important for me to see that the feelings and reactions we were keeping to ourselves were preventing us from going anywhere. I learned that conflict that isn't brought out into the open doesn't magically disappear. And I saw that expressing this conflict was all right."

By allowing every member to share significant moments and lessons, this technique helps bring the entire group experience back to all the members. People have a chance to see how their work had an influence on others. The leader can help the conceptualization process by asking members what they learned about themselves and others during these significant moments. This technique of recalling and sharing events is generally a special time and a valuable experience.

Expressing negative aspects of a group experience. Typically, as a group nears termination, we ask members to clear the air regarding aspects of the group that they might go away viewing negatively. We worry that group members will put on a false, positive front at the end of a group but will later nurse grievances that they never noticed. We may express our usual warning that what you don't say may often be more harmful than what you do say. We do not especially encourage members to say harsh things to one another at the very end of a group, when there is no opportunity to follow up or work through replies, but we do ask them to be forthright with us, even in the final phase, concerning any features of the group experience about which they are critical. Having made every effort to encourage the voicing of the negative, we hope that the group members will leave their experience with a generally positive opinion and that they will have stated their gains in ways that will help to make these memorable and lasting.

Techniques for bringing out the negative might include the following:

- "Suppose it's a year from now and you're sitting around with some buddies. The conversation turns to derogatory remarks about therapy groups. What can you imagine yourself saying? Is it likely that you might join in and describe groups such as this in a negative way?" Here the leader might allude to complaints that have come up during the life of the group. "Might you complain that these experiences aren't really genuine and lasting?

Might you you complain that people felt forced to talk about problems they didn't want to discuss?"

- "Imagine yourself driving home awhile from now. What might you be thinking about this group? Maybe you'll have in mind something about how the group has been conducted that isn't so positive and that you're perhaps feeling but not saying right now."
- "As well as reviewing the highlights of this group, we might want to take some time to reflect on the moments that weren't so good. Where were some junctures that you had your doubts about all this?"
- "Suppose it's a year from now, and you have gone into individual therapy. You're telling your therapist about features of this group experience that you believe were counterproductive for you. Would you be willing to tell us a bit about what complaints come to mind?"

Exploring the issue of separation. As members terminate an ongoing group, separation becomes a particularly critical issue. As we mentioned earlier, both the member who is terminating and those who are remaining need a chance to express the meaning of what they have shared.

In the case of a closed group, particularly if it has become a cohesive unit, the members commonly feel resistance over leaving. They are often concerned that they will not be as open and trusting with people outside the group. They wonder whether they will experience the same closeness, caring, nonjudgmental atmosphere, and support once they leave the group. Although leaders cannot deny the importance of recognizing and exploring the feelings of members about separation, they can also encourage members to look for support in their relationships outside the group. Leaders might remind members that the closeness they value in the group did not happen by accident. Clients need to recognize what they did to create this special climate. They need to recall that they made a commitment to create an effective group and that they initiated trust. They can then consider how to continue reaching out in similar ways in everyday situations.

Rehearsing new roles. Role-playing techniques can be extremely effective in giving people a chance to practice new behaviors. Of course, the process of rehearsing new roles ought to occur at all the stages of a group, not just during its final phase. Through the technique of rehearsing alternative roles, members can receive feedback from others in the group on the impact they might have, and others can provide alternative behaviors that they may not have thought of.

A common mistake of some participants is to focus on how they might change others in their lives rather than on what they might change about themselves. Leaders can stress that members have the power to change themselves but cannot directly change others. In the group, for example, Al became aware that he had been holding most of his feelings of both anger and tenderness within himself. He learned that expressing feelings was not unmanly and that terrible consequences didn't follow when he did express himself. Al is now concerned for his children, whom he sees as holding in their feelings. During a role rehearsal he lectures them about the benefits of expressing emotions. In their feedback the other members remind Al that his children are more likely to begin to express their feelings if he expresses his own emotions to them rather than telling them why they should do so.

Some other members also become impatient with their loved ones, wanting them to share the level of awareness they have reached through their group experience. They forget that they had to work to achieve that awareness. After they role-play the situations they expect to encounter, other members may remind them that their impatience and insistence on instant change will push people away. It is important to continually remind participants that they are in a group to change themselves, not others. People have a better chance to control themselves and to decide how they will change, but they run into trouble when they decide how others ought to be different from them.

Another common pitfall for people leaving a group is that they often come to rely on group jargon. Even within the group people may lose a full awareness of their concerns when they rely too much on expressions like "staying with your feelings," "projecting," and "getting away from 'shoulds.' " And members are likely to alienate people outside the group if they use such language. Role-playing conversations that they intend to have with others can help them overcome this tendency.

Being specific about outcomes and plans. During all group sessions members should avoid general and global statements and instead be specific and descriptive. During the final stage of a group, being specific is especially important if members are to be clear about what they learned about themselves and how they are going to apply these lessons. If a member says "This group has been very good for me—I've learned a lot and grown a lot," the leader's response might be: "Specifically, what did you learn, and how did you see yourself as growing? In what ways has this group been good for you? What are some things that have been good for you?" If members are specific both about what they have learned and about their plans for change, the likelihood that they will act to change their behavior is increased.

Feedback during the final stage also needs to be specific. Members can be discouraged from categorizing others as they give feedback and from saying something they have not said to others before in the group, especially something negative. Introducing new material is not helpful at this time, when the point is to consolidate what has already been seen. A final feedback session is not an opportunity to attack someone or to hit and run, nor is it the time to shower someone with such syrupy sweetness that the person has a hyperglycemic reaction! During the final feedback session, what is valuable are specific reactions, impressions, and brief comments. One technique is to ask the people receiving feedback not to respond but to listen carefully to what is being said. Their silence does not imply that they accept the feedback as valid. It simply helps them consider what they hear more seriously than they might if they were to give an immediate response.

Another feedback procedure is to ask members to finish some of the following incomplete statements for each participant:

- "My fear for you is . . ."
- "My hope for you is . . ."
- "What I'd like for you to remember most is . . ."
- "One thing I like best about you is . . ."
- "One thing that distances you from me is . . ."
- "A way I see you as blocking your strengths is . . ."

Another member can write down the comments for each person receiving feedback and then give the person these notes. Or members can write down their sentence completions and then give them to each participant. This procedure makes forgetting these comments less likely.

Projecting the future. The leader can ask members to think of the changes they would most like to have made six months hence, one year hence, and five years hence. Members can then imagine that the entire group is meeting at one of these designated times and can say what they'd most want to say to the others at that time. They can also outline what they will have to do to accomplish these goals. This device focuses members on the changes they'd like to make in their lives on both a short-term and a long-term basis.

Members sometimes express the fear that they will not change. Here a useful technique is to ask them to imagine meeting again one year later and to express their feelings about changes they haven't made: "How do you feel about continuing pretty much as you were a year ago, when the group ended?" If they say that they would feel pretty dismal, the leaders can challenge them to develop an action plan for change. They could say any of the following: "What are just a few steps that you're willing to commit to so that you'll move in the direction you want?" "What is it that you see you need to do at this time so that you won't wind up disappointed?" "Are there any people in this group whom you're willing to call once the group has ended?"

Summarizing personal reactions to the group. During the last session of a group it's valuable for members to make at least brief statements about what it was like for them to be members and to summarize what they are taking with them as a result of the experience. Again, the rationale is that members will carry away more information from a group if they verbalize their reactions and give meaning and perspective to what they've learned. Here are some examples of questions that members might address:

- "What has it been like for you to be a member of this group? What have you liked or disliked about being in the group?"
- "What have you learned about yourself? What did you learn about how others view you?"

- "What were some of the major turning points in this group for you? What were a few of the most significant events for you?"
- "What are some of the things you most want to say as this group is closing?"

This technique allows all members to have some idea of what each person is taking away from the group. It also encourages members to think through and to pull together the lessons they have learned.

Making contracts.   Making contracts to carry out further action once the group ends can be a valuable way to help members try new behaviors in their day-to-day living. One technique is to ask members to bring a written statement about a change they are willing to make once the group ends. Participants can read their contracts aloud, and others can give specific suggestions for fulfilling the contracts and can comment on the degree to which the contracts seem realistic.

David, for example, has come to realize through his group work that he consistently puts himself down with self-defeating remarks and does not try new activities for fear of failure. He knows that he is setting himself up for failure with his internal dialogue. He decides that he wants to change this behavior by attempting new projects. He lists several of these projects and asks the group to suggest how he can avoid slipping back into his old ways. As a result of their suggestions, he agrees as part of his contract to make several signs and tape them to the mirror in his bathroom, to the refrigerator door, and in other places in the house. The signs read: "I have a right to ask for what I want." "I don't have to continue to set myself up for defeat." "I can and will do more than I've told myself I could do in the past."

Learning not to discount or forget.   Members tend to forget what they've learned in a group or to discount the insights they've had. After the termination of a group, members may tell themselves that the group experience cannot be replicated in everyday life. For example, Loretta convinces herself that people in the group were just being kind to her and that she cannot find the same support for making changes now that she has left the group.

In the discounting exercise, several members form an inner circle and talk as if they were meeting several months after the termination of the group. They speak particularly about all the ways in which they might be lessening the value of the group and discounting their experience. The rationale is to give members a chance to foresee the internal dialogue they might engage in as time moves on. Alternatively, they can role-play how they might depreciate their group experience when describing it to people in their everyday lives. If members are thus confronted with the likelihood of forgetting and discounting, they are less likely to do so.

Techniques for Continuing Assessment and Follow Up

Ethical considerations in evaluation and follow up. Part of effective practice entails developing strategies to ensure continuing assessment and designing follow-up procedures for a group. Below are some specific recommendations of the ASGW to keep in mind when designing follow-up and evaluation strategies:

- Group counselors recognize the importance of ongoing assessment of a group, and they assist members in evaluating their own progress.
- Group counselors conduct evaluation of the total group experience at the final meeting (or before termination), as well as ongoing evaluation.
- Group counselors monitor their own behavior and become aware of what they are modeling in the group.
- Follow-up procedures might take the form of personal contact, telephone contact, or written contact.
- Follow-up meetings might be with individuals, or groups, or both to determine the degree to which: i) members have reached their goals, (ii) the group had a positive or negative effect on the participants, (iii) members could profit from some type of referral, and (iv) as information for possible modification of future groups [*sic*]. If there is no follow-up meeting, provisions are made available for individual follow-up meetings to any member who needs or requests such a contact.

Conducting follow-up interviews. As a safety check and as a method of assessment, leaders can try to arrange a private interview with each group member a few weeks to a few months after the group ends. Such an interview can be beneficial to the client as a "booster shot" and can also provide a measure of the group's effectiveness.

The purpose of this session is to determine the degree to which members have met their personal goals and fulfilled their contracts. It's a chance for both leaders and members to discuss the impact of the group, to talk about specific ways of continuing whatever learning was begun, and to discuss any unfinished business or feelings left over from the group. If members are having problems using what they learned, this individual contact is an opportunity to explore ways of dealing with these difficulties. It is also an excellent opportunity for leaders to suggest other groups or individual counseling if it seems appropriate.

Encouraging contact with other members. A technique that can lend support to members as they are practicing new behavior or completing an action program is to periodically contact another member from the group after termination. This contact can be especially important when members find that they are not pushing themselves to do much now that the group has finished. By calling another member and reporting on their progress or lack of it, they can gain both support and stimulation. Members can select one or more persons with whom they are willing to make contact for at least a few months after termination to report progress toward their goals. This is a method of accountability, and it is a way for people to learn how to establish a support system.

Arranging a follow-up session.   A follow-up session can take place a couple of months after the end of the group to assess the impact of the group on each of the members. Having such a session is one more way of maximizing the chance that members will receive lasting benefit from the group experience. Because members know that they will meet with the group at some future time to review what they've done, they are more likely to stick to their contracts. We stress in our groups how crucial it is that all members attend the follow-up, regardless of whether they have stuck to their plan for change. Sometimes members who feel that they have let themselves down by not having done what they promised may be tempted to "forget" about the follow-up or to claim that they are "too busy." We emphasize that they can learn a great deal from one another by sharing the difficulties they encountered in using what they had learned in the group once they no longer had its support. Such a session also provides a chance for them to acknowledge how the lessons they learned fit their lives, and the leader can get a sense of the overall impact of the group.

Suggesting where to go for further growth.   A group experience may be just the beginning of growth for many of the members. Even though some members may appear to get little from their first group, it often readies them for future growth experiences. Thus, during the final session, the follow-up interview, or the follow-up session, leaders can give a number of suggestions to those participants who wish to continue the work they've begun. These suggestions may include specific recommendations for individual counseling and therapy and recommendations for other closed groups, workshops, or perhaps an ongoing group with some of the same members from the group that just terminated. Leaders can also suggest reading material and perhaps organizations that members can contact for a variety of social activities. The members themselves might use part of the final session to brainstorm about ways of going further with their work. Because members may be ready to consider another group or individual counseling only after some time has elapsed, the follow-up session is an excellent place to reinforce the value of getting involved in various growth projects.

Techniques for Evaluating a Group

Evaluation form.   Leaders can use some type of assessment device to determine the outcomes of a group. We favor devices that tap the subjective reactions of the members both at the final session and at the follow-up session.

There is often a significant difference in how members feel about a group immediately after it ends and how they feel several months later. Feedback in both instances is valuable.

An evaluation form can ask members to assess their degree of satisfaction with the group and the level of investment they had in it; to recall highlights or significant events; to specify actions they took during the group to make desired changes; to specify what techniques were most and least helpful and to suggest changes in the format; and to describe how the group appears through their eyes after some time has elapsed. Depending on the membership, a structured checklist might be devised, an open-ended letter might be asked for, or a combination of a rating scale and essay questions might be used.

This evaluation procedure is valuable not only as a way for leaders to measure the effectiveness of the group but also as a way for the members to focus their thinking on what they did during the group and what they received from the experience. The questionnaire below is one evaluation form that leaders can use to get some idea of the impact of the group on the members.

• •

Member Evaluation Form

1. What general effect has your group experience had on your life?
2. What were the highlights of the group experience for you?
3. What specific things did you become aware of about yourself—about your lifestyle, attitudes, and relationships with others?
4. What changes have you made in your life that you can attribute at least partially to your group experience?
5. Which of the techniques used by the group leaders had the most impact on you? Which techniques had the least impact?
6. What are some of your perceptions of the group leaders and their styles?
7. What problems did you encounter in the outside world when you tried to carry out some of the decisions you made in the group?
8. What are some of the questions you have asked yourself since the group ended?
9. Did the group experience have any negative effects on you?
10. Is there anything about groups in general, about this group, or about how it was conducted that you find yourself viewing critically or negatively?
11. How did your participation in the group affect significant people in your life?
12. How might your life be different if you had not been a member of the group?
13. If you had to say in a sentence or two what the group meant to you, how would you respond?

• •

Group leader's journal.   As we recommended earlier, keeping a journal is an excellent idea for both group members and group leaders. For leaders, it helps them evaluate the progress of a group and assess changes during the stages of its development. They can focus not only on what occurs within the group and on the members' behavior but also on their own reactions. Here are some areas that leaders might write about:

- How did you initially view the group? What were your reactions to the group as a whole?
- What were some initial reactions you had to each member? How did any of these reactions or impressions change? What members did you find yourself most wanting to work with? What members did you have difficulty with?
- How did you feel in leading this group? Did you generally want to be in the group? Did you take your share of responsibility for the group's progress?
- Were there any times that you felt stuck with the group because of a personal concern that you have not explored? Did you find yourself avoiding certain topics because of your own discomfort with these topics?
- What turning points did you see in this group?
- What factors do you see as contributing to the success or failure of the group?
- How open were you to taking and considering nondefensively the feedback you received from the members?
- What techniques did you use, and what were the outcomes?
- What were the key events of each session?
- Describe the dynamics of the group and the relationships among members.
- If this group were composed of members very much like yourself, what kind of group do you think it would have been?
- What did you learn about yourself from leading this group?
- What lessons can you learn from the reactions you had toward specific members?

By keeping such a journal, you can review trends in the group and devise changes in format or techniques for future groups.

You might also type up your observations of each session and give these notes to the members before the following session. Members, too, can be encouraged to keep brief process journals, and you and the members can share your observations. At termination, these journals provide a summary of significant events in the group. In addition, when co-leaders meet to discuss the group's progress, they can refer to their process notes for any differences in perceptions.

Finally, this journal is a good device for generating personal work for you as a leader. You can reserve a section of the journal for writing down whatever comes to mind about unresolved problems in your life. For example, if you become aware of hurt feelings and rejection through the work of some members, you may choose not to work on that problem in the group itself but can profit from writing in your journal about further work that you might do in your own therapy.

Concluding Comments

In this chapter we have emphasized the importance of ending sessions and terminating groups in such a way as to maximize learning and provide an opportunity for growth and change. Reviewing highlights, consolidating lessons, role playing, getting and giving feedback, and writing are all useful techniques during the final stage. A group will not promote insight or growth if the leader fails to pay sufficient attention to its ending phases or emphasizes just the experiential dimension of the group process without enlisting the intellects of members to give meaning to what they have experienced.

Questions and Activities

1. Suppose that your group is almost at the end of a session and several people introduce new and potent material. What might you say or do in response? Can you think of any ways in which you might have set the members up to introduce new material at the end?
2. Describe some techniques or strategies that you might employ to wrap up a particular session of a group.
3. We have said that not acknowledging a group's termination may reflect an unconscious desire on the part of the leaders or members to avoid dealing with separation and endings. How might your own feelings and reactions toward the termination of a group that you are leading affect the manner in which members fully explore their own feelings about the group's termination?
4. Describe what you regard as the most important gains from group work and how the ending of a session can enhance these gains. Discuss variables such as the group's population and its stated purpose.
5. What value do you see in homework assignments and other suggestions for action that are designed to give members practice in new behavior outside group sessions? What techniques of this kind might you use in one of your groups?
6. Suppose a member of your group comments on your looking at your watch. What might you say? As a group leader, do you pay attention to time, and do you allow sufficient time at the end of a session for a summary and integration of what has taken place? What are some techniques that you might employ in this regard?
7. When and how might you reintroduce material that a member of your group worked on in a previous session? What are some important considerations here? Would you remind a member of something she seemed

to have left unfinished at the prior session? If she indicated that she could no longer get into it, then what would you do?

8. What are some issues you'd want to consider when terminating an open group? a closed group?

9. At the last meeting of a ten-week group, several members urge you to extend the group for a few weeks. What theoretical considerations seem significant to you in this situation? How would you deal with this matter?

10. The group has come to an end, and a member expresses an interest in continuing in a social relationship with you. What considerations do you think are especially important here?

11. We discuss some techniques for having members review significant moments in the group's history. Invent some similar techniques of your own, and imagine how they might go.

12. A supervisor asks you how your group is going. What criteria would you use in replying?

13. We suggest some questions to use on an assessment form for having members evaluate a session. Write an assessment form that would be suitable for a group you might lead. Why would you or wouldn't you use such a form?

14. What are the most important considerations during the final stage of a group? What specific issues would you want members of your group to focus on during this phase, and what techniques could you use to help them do so?

15. A member plans to leave a group that will continue to meet. How do you see this sort of termination as different from the termination of the whole group? What issues are different?

16. Members cannot possibly remember everything they experience in a group. What would you most hope that participants would remember, and what techniques might you use to help them recall and review these lessons?

17. What negative consequences do you think there might be if members do not deal explicitly with the fact that the group is ending? What techniques might you use if you sense participants are inclined to avoid talking about the group's termination?

18. Toward the end of a group you ask the members to talk about what they have gained from the experience. One of them says: "I really have gotten a lot from this. I've experienced different things, and I've gotten in touch with my feelings. It was great!" Would you have any concerns about this person's remarks, and what might you say to him?

19. We have said that transfer of learning from the group to everyday life does not happen automatically—that it should be fostered and structured. What are your thoughts on this topic? What techniques would facilitate transferring what was learned in the group to other situations?

20. Imagine planning with a colleague or a fellow student strategies to use during the final few sessions before your group ends. If you are opposed to planning strategies in advance, explain why.

21. Your group is holding a follow-up session several months after its termination. What questions would you most want to ask the participants? What do you see as the significant goals of this meeting?

22. Follow-up sessions may lead participants to feel guilty about progress they have not made. What techniques could you use to enhance the gains that people did make?

23. What are some ways in which you would attempt to evaluate the outcomes of your groups?

24. You suggest to a participant that taking part in another group or in individual counseling might be a good idea for her. She says she feels that you are telling her that she has failed to get anything from your group. What might you say to her? What referrals might you make, or what ideas for further group or individual counseling might you suggest to members in general?

25. We discussed the value of group leaders' keeping a journal in which they write process notes as well as describe their personal reactions. What value do you see such a journal having in helping you assess a group's progress? What specific topics do you think you'd most want to include in your process journal? Discuss.

CHAPTER EIGHT

In a Nutshell

In this chapter we isolate and highlight a series of points that clarify some of the underlying principles of our style of leadership. We want to emphasize that these are our views and that we are presenting them for you to consider and to adapt for yourself in a way that makes sense. This list should not be read as a series of dogmatic pronouncements about the best way to lead a group. These are simply ideas that have worked for us.

Recognize the primacy of the client. In this book we may have seemed more directive and structured in our leadership style than is really the case. Perhaps that impression was unavoidable, given that the book is about techniques. Although we take an active role in leading, we see ourselves as constantly responding to our clients and seeking to flow with them. We see therapy as a kind of dance: sometimes we lead and sometimes we follow, but in either case we try to be aware of how we can best move with our partners. Sensitivity to and respect for clients are fundamental to the therapeutic interaction. We seek to suit techniques to clients rather than molding them to our needs and our techniques.

Put aside prejudices and assumptions. If you want to be a therapeutic agent, you must put aside your preconceived notions about the people with whom you work. It is critical that you develop an awareness of the negative impact of stereotyping individuals because of their age, disability, ethnicity, gender, race, religion, or sexual preference. Try to avoid making assumptions about clients, and be open to letting them tell you who they are and what is important to them. In this way you can avoid imposing your values and your vision of reality on clients who differ from you. Your techniques will certainly take into account factors such as the client's age and cultural background. For example, if you are working with adolescents and introduce a technique that assumes they feel rebellious, or if you are working with the elderly and introduce a technique that assumes they are no longer sexual, you are imposing your preconceived notions rather than allowing your clients to tell you who they are.

Adapt your techniques to the needs of culturally diverse clients. Since culture does influence a client's behavior, whether or not the group counselor is aware of it, responsible and effective practice entails an understanding of the range of cultural similarities and differences. It is useful to consider culture from a broad perspective that includes factors such as ethnicity, family traditions and beliefs, religion, race, socioeconomic status, and gender. It is essential that you discover ways to modify your strategies to meet the unique needs of a group composed of culturally diverse members. Your genuine respect for the differences among members in your groups will be the most important foundation on which to build a bridge between yourself and them. Effective multicultural practice demands an open stance on your part and a flexibility in adapting your techniques to fit the needs and situations of the individuals within the group. No one "right" set of techniques can be utilized across the board, irrespective of a client's cultural background.

Be aware of values. We have said that techniques are an extension of you as a person but are also created to fit the context and the character of the client. It is not possible for your own values, which are a part of your character, to be excluded from the material you pursue and the techniques you suggest. Strive to develop an awareness of how your values and needs are likely to influence the interventions you make. Although ethical practice dictates that you take care to avoid *imposing* your values on members, it is important that you *expose* your beliefs, values, and needs in cases where concealing them is likely to create problems for those who participate in your groups.

Our own experience in group work shows us that the techniques we create are often a reflection of the values we hold. There are times when, in suggesting a technique, we imply the direction in which we want group members to try to go. When we propose a new behavior, we are indicating that this behavior is one we hope our clients might incorporate. For example, if we encourage a client to role-play striking up a conversation with a member of the opposite sex, we are hoping that the client can learn to be more comfortable doing so. The fact that our techniques reflect our values does not mean that we are imposing these values on the group. The fact that we have hopes for how our clients might become does not mean that we do not respect them for reaching their own decisions. Generally, we take our cues from what our clients indicate they want for themselves. When our own values come into play, we feel that at least we can be aware of them in ourselves. If a value of yours is that conflict should be avoided at all costs, you are likely to introduce techniques that bypass conflict. If a value of yours is that anger needs to be expressed, you are likely to develop techniques for dealing with the expression of anger. Minimally, you can be aware of your preferences and can make yourself and your values known to clients. In that way you are not as likely to use your preferences to manipulate others.

Realize the importance of preparation. It is a good practice to prepare both yourself and the members for a group experience. Adequate preparation reduces the risks of group work and maximizes effectiveness. Much of what goes wrong in some groups and much of what accounts for why they never reach an effective working stage can be traced to the lack of an adequate foundation. Preparation includes informing potential members about the nature of the group, teaching them about how they might get the most from a group experience, and encouraging them to focus on the specific issues and concerns they wish to explore. You can get yourself psychologically ready for a group by taking time to reflect on your own life and to think about your objectives for the group. Preparing with a co-leader whom you can learn from and who complements your own style can be ideal.

Emphasize confidentiality. Group participants are not going to reveal themselves in meaningful ways unless they feel quite sure that they can trust both you and the other members to respect what they share. One of your key responsibilities as a group leader is to protect members by defining clearly what confidentiality means and helping them understand the difficulties involved in maintaining it. Of course, the limitations of confidentiality are an issue that needs to be clarified at the outset, such as those situations in which you are legally obliged to divulge confidences. At appropriate times throughout a group, you might remind the members how crucial maintaining confidentiality is to their effective work.

Although members will inevitably want to talk about their group experiences with significant people in their life, it is wise to caution them about the subtle ways in which they might unintentionally violate others' confidences in this process. As a general rule, members do not violate confidentiality when they talk about *what* they learned about themselves in a group. They tend to get into trouble when they begin to talk about *how* others made changes by describing what others did or what techniques were used.

Use techniques as means, not ends. Techniques are no better than the person using them and are no good at all if they are not sensitively adapted to the particular client and context. The outcome of a technique is affected by the climate of the group and by the relationship between therapist and client. Techniques are a means to an end; they amplify material that is present and encourage exploration of where that material is leading. If you become more concerned with techniques than with your capacity to dance with your clients, or if techniques become ends in themselves, the heart of the group process has been lost.

Cultivate the soil. Techniques should not be sprung on group members or be imposed without regard for the degree to which a relationship with the members has been cultivated. Particularly with techniques that evoke intense emotion, we seek to gauge the readiness of the client to work with us and with the exercise we are proposing. Instead of commanding, we invite clients to experiment and allow them to disagree. It is our task to earn their trust by demonstrating our goodwill.

Use tentative language. We characteristically introduce a technique by saying "I wonder whether you would be willing to . . . ," "How would it be if you . . . ," or "Do you suppose you could . . . ?" When we offer an interpretation, we typically begin by saying "I have a hunch that . . ." or "If I were you, I might feel that . . ." We try in our choice of words not to give the impression that we are pronouncing unimpeachable diagnoses from on high. We do not, however, water our words down with meaningless qualifiers.

We give our own confrontive feedback, for example, in a direct and un-qualified way. But in providing interpretations and in introducing techniques, we employ tentative language that gives the client room to gracefully decline.

Use simple language. We introduce techniques so simply and clearly that a child could understand the instructions. Groups inevitably develop their own special language and metaphors, but we tend to discourage using over-worked popular expressions and psychobabble like "getting in touch with your feelings." We strive to use language that is clear and descriptive.

Be aware of nonverbal communication. We seek to be conscious of the nonverbal communications of the clients and of how we nonverbally pre-sent ourselves to the group. In order to establish a trusting relationship, we choose our words to communicate a basic respect for the people we work with. We recognize the importance of paying attention not only to the con-tent of a member's speech but also to the manner in which the client presents messages. We look for patterns of nonverbal communications, yet we gener-ally avoid quickly interpreting the meaning underlying these messages. In-stead, we ask clients to become aware of their own body language and other nonverbal forms of communication and to attach their own meanings to pat-terns that emerge within the group.

Present the problem to the group. Group leaders often wonder how to handle a situation and fail to utilize the most obvious resource: the wisdom of the group members. One of the simplest ways to get good help from the members is to ask for it, to present the problem to them. For instance, if we are trying to think of a technique that might enhance a member's direc-tion or are wondering how to modify a technique that is going nowhere, we may simply state the problem as we see it to the group and ask for sug-gestions. These interjections do double duty: they serve as interpretations or clarifications, and they constructively involve the group members in the process of seeking solutions.

Don't fight the river. We may sometimes introduce a technique with a preconceived idea of what is going to happen, but the material that emerges may lead in another direction. Or a client may misunderstand our directions and do something quite different from what we had in mind. We also find that a technique may work well once or many times, but we can't always count on its working the same way twice. There are times when we have a sense of what we would like to introduce into a session, such as a focus on a particular theme or topic, yet the group may show little interest in pur-suing our agenda. In all these instances, we prefer not to fight the river. A lesson that we continue to relearn is to "go with the flow."

Be willing to experiment. In some ways the difference between an ex-perienced leader and an inexperienced one lies in a willingness to experi-ment and to forge ahead. We find that we can't draw on our capacity for spontaneously utilizing our own emotional resources if we are afraid to ex-periment in creating techniques to fit a context. We teach beginning group leaders to be aware of certain pitfalls and to take necessary precautions, but we equally seek to encourage them to trust themselves. If you find yourself becoming stale or uncreative, you might consider getting more supervision, working more with different co-leaders, or attending different sorts of workshops as a participant.

Be willing to seek consultation. There will be times when you can profit from the input of colleagues, supervisors, or other professionals. Ethical practice involves the willingness to seek appropriate professional assistance when you become aware that your own personal problems or conflicts are likely to impair your professional judgment and your work with clients. Additionally, it is a mark of your professionalism to seek out consultation or supervision regarding ethical concerns when you encounter difficulties that interfere with your effectiveness in carrying out leadership functions.

Realize that therapy is necessary for yourself. As a group counselor, you should recognize that exploring your own life is a long-term commitment. You probably cannot, and, in any case should not, take your clients any further than you yourself are willing to go. To some degree we find that our own therapy deepens and progresses as a consequence of leading, but we believe it important to make periodic efforts to explore ourselves further. One interesting way to gauge the progress of your own therapy is to ask yourself these questions: "Realistically, what would a group be like if it were composed of members whose personalities were like mine? Where would such a group bog down? What kinds of resistance would tend to emerge in it?"

Link the work of clients. For exercises to be genuinely group techniques, they generally ought to allow for several members to work at the same time. Some individual work in a group setting can be fine, but involving several clients better utilizes time and resources. In this area the leader orchestrates the group using creativity and intuition to identify common themes from the information that clients have provided and to indicate how members can work together on these themes.

Use props. We find that techniques can be considerably enriched if we pay attention to useful items in the immediate environment. In working with a client who spoke of feeling boxed in we saw a large cardboard box outside. After the box was brought into the room, the client got inside and spoke about the various things that he felt were closing him in. Such employment of props can enhance techniques that seek to magnify an experience and can provide clients with valuable symbols in their subsequent reflections.

Use the client's metaphors. We have emphasized throughout this book that we try to follow the lead provided by our group members' material and that we see techniques as a means of enhancing what is going on rather than trying to generate a direction according to our own agenda. A key aspect of this view is that we invent techniques that utilize the phrasings and metaphors introduced by the group member. The member's language finds its way into our ideas for techniques, and it provides us with the occasion for creative work.

In supervising student group leaders, we find that, out of anxiety, they tend to focus on the client's literal message. They actually do not hear the member's metaphor, or if they do, they often do not appreciate the rich source of meaning contained in it. For example, when members say that they feel empty inside, it is therapeutically useful to look beyond the literal by encouraging them to explore what emptiness means to them. How do they describe emptiness? How do they experience emptiness? If they feel empty, what may they be missing? What are they inclined to do with this feeling?

Consider the richness of the following metaphors: "I feel that I spilled my guts, and now I'm left hanging." "Whenever I open my mouth in here, I expect to get pounced on." "I made myself vulnerable in here, and I feel as if I've been sliced to bits." "I feel like a piece of meat that has been through a meat grinder." Any of these symbols speaks volumes about the experience of a member. For instance, it would be interesting to pursue who is the "meat" and who is "grinding" it. If members are willing to talk about their honest reactions, there is a good chance that the group will become a safer place that will allow for productive work. Members have a lot to express through their metaphors, and leaders need to understand the deeper meaning of the members' words.

Create techniques to fit the context. We see our principal role as following the material introduced by the members and opening these issues up for exploration, rather than attempting to find solutions to problems. We try to use techniques that facilitate the flow of topics and are adapted to them and that highlight connections between topics and links between members.

Use humor. Although humor can be used to deflect painful or uncomfortable situations in a group, if used appropriately and timed well, it can also be therapeutic. We have often been struck by how clients can laugh about topics they were crying over only a few minutes before. We don't hesitate to have fun and to make humor part of the techniques we introduce. For genuine and constructive humor to be used in a group, we find, there has to be a strong level of trust. Furthermore, humor should never be used to denigrate a member. In a climate of respect the humor involves laughing *with* members, not *at* them.

Go with the obvious. Although we may use complex interpretations as a way of thinking about our clients, we want to work with what is present and obvious. There are times, when a group seems flat, that you might be tempted to assume responsibility by using techniques to "get the group going." Rather than trying to bring energy to the group, we suggest that you call attention to what is happening. Try to think of ways of using techniques that will accentuate what is obvious.

Think about theory. We emphasize the importance of continually rethinking our theoretical orientations. A theory is a cognitive map, but not a fixed map. Our theories about how we work are open to modifications based on experience. At any given time we are able to say how we are viewing human nature and how this view affects our style of therapy, what our rationale is for introducing the techniques we do, and what our vision is of what we have to offer clients. Many practitioners have a high regard for their intuitions and hunches but an aversion to the intellect and an unwillingness to reflect on what they are doing. If techniques are to be extensions of the therapist's character, leaders must be willing to frequently review their theoretical assumptions.

Recognize the limits of responsibility. We see the therapeutic partnership as a shared examination of our lives, our feelings, and our possibilities for being different. Earlier, we used the metaphor of therapy as a dance, in which the therapist sometimes leads, sometimes follows, but always seeks to go with the shared movement. Responsibility for the success of the dance is not ours alone. We see our responsibilities primarily as preparing ourselves and our members for the group experience, providing a context in which meaningful work is likely to occur, making ourselves available to hear and encounter our clients, providing skills and techniques that facilitate the explorations of the group, and seeking to maximize the opportunity to learn from the experience. If a group goes well, it is not all to our credit, and if a group is unproductive, it is not all our fault.

Don't attempt to change people directly. We assume that our clients may change profoundly under our influence, but we don't see these changes as something we do to them as if they, like the sculptor's clay, were the passive recipients of our technical manipulations. We do not think that people's lives simply and passively undergo transformation as a result of what we do. We seek to provide an optimal environment, or context, within which group participants can express what they feel, reexamine and rethink decisions they have made, try out new behavior, and, in short, consider how they could change. Although a technique we introduce can invite participants to change and encourage them to do so, we do not think it is the technique that brings the change about. The technique simply enhances the client's awareness of the possibility of being different. Once the client is aware of these options, the hardest work begins as the client attempts to carry what has been learned into daily life.

Attempt to integrate thinking, feeling, and doing. People cannot be segmented, because thinking, feeling, and acting are necessarily interdependent. One dimension of human functioning invariably affects other aspects of behavior. Thus, our techniques work better when we strive to utilize all modes of experience. If we sometimes ask clients to refrain from thinking about what they are saying, our goal is to have them eventually think clearly and be in a position to change. Some theories of therapy emphasize feeling as opposed to thinking; some stress thinking rather than feeling; some accentuate behavior independently of thinking or feeling. Our style of leadership and the techniques we employ emphasize the integration of these three dimensions. We seek through our use of techniques to give our clients an opportunity to experience and express their emotions. But we are also concerned to have them reflect on how their feelings connect with their belief systems, the assumptions they make, and the early decisions on which these assumptions may be based. We focus considerably on what they are currently doing, realizing that their actions are influenced by what they are thinking and feeling. Then we encourage them to try out different ways of behaving within the group and, lastly, to consider ways of carrying concrete behavioral changes into their lives outside the group.

Encourage verbalization. A great many of our techniques emphasize verbal behavior: role playing, sentence completions, and go-arounds. This emphasis fits with our theoretical commitment to thinking, feeling, and doing as a package, because what we say reveals how we think, feel, and act. Typically, when we ask group members to say something, our hope is to promote their talking spontaneously and unguardedly. Contrary to popular group jargon, we are not exactly seeking to have our clients "get out of their heads" or "turn off their intellects." However, we are asking them to refrain from being too guarded by being overly cerebral. By the same token, talking differently is one way of being different. Techniques that ask clients to say something different explore the possibility of change, pointing to how they could think, feel, and act.

Explore polarities. To achieve our goal of integrating thinking, feeling, and doing, we seek to acknowledge and work with polarities in our clients. All clients have opposite sides within them, even though they often do not want to acknowledge or own them: a thinking side versus a feeling side, being like one parent versus being like the other, being dependent versus being independent, being passive versus being active, being trusting versus being suspicious, and being open versus being closed. Many of our techniques ask group members to exaggerate one side of themselves in order to stay with it long enough to get more information about it and to decide whether it is a way they want to be. Our techniques do not aim at getting rid of one side. Rather, we find that having clients acknowledge various sides of themselves through techniques that emphasize polarities is a prelude to their accepting parts of themselves that they have needlessly rejected, rejecting parts they have needlessly accepted, and considering possibilities for integrated change.

Work with the past, present, and future. Some leaders think of their groups as having a present, or here-and-now, orientation, whereas others focus on the past. In a way, one of our biggest concerns is to devise techniques that focus on the future, on how clients could be. However, the groundwork for change is getting clients clear about who they are now, based on their personal histories. Our techniques move back and forth among all three temporal frames of reference. Typically, we begin with current concerns introduced by group members and with dynamics we see in the group. We assume that present material is rooted in childhood lessons, but when we introduce techniques that focus on the past, we seek to use only material that can be made experientially present. We also operate on the assumption that if we focus on the client's present state, this person's unfinished business from the past will become evident. There are themes in a person's life, and we are interested in seeing connections between one's past and one's current personality. To make the past more relevant and to explore it in a more lively way, we frequently ask clients to bring their past into the present by imagining and reliving significant scenarios. We may ask: "If you could be that hurt child who you were then, what would you want people to know about you? What would you want from them?" "What do you want to say now to your father that you didn't say then?" "Could you exaggerate a part of you that you learned from your mother as a child?" We avoid exploring past history in an abstract and detached way. We seek to examine the relevance of the past by reliving it and connecting it with current struggles. The point of such techniques is to put clients into a position to choose how they want to be now in light of their beginnings.

Be aware of the ethical context. There are risks specifically related to group techniques, but they can be minimized. As you will recall, it is critical to adequately prepare members to derive the maximum benefit from a group. Techniques should be genuinely geared to further the goals of the members rather than being artifically imposed. We encourage you not to hide behind techniques but to base your interventions on a theoretical framework that you are developing.

Provide opportunities to consolidate learning and to practice new behavior. The final stage of a group presents an ideal opportunity for using techniques that enable members to remember the specifics of their group experience, to seek a cognitive framework for lessons they want to take away, to practice new behavior, and to deal with the emotional significance of termination. This stage is important if the group is to be more than a passing experience. Ideally, it should promote consolidation, generalization, and transfer of learning.

Learn to dance with clients. Group techniques cannot be an artificial substitute for a therapeutic and human encounter between you and the members who trust you to facilitate their group. Techniques can creatively invigorate this encounter and give form to its expression, however, when you learn to dance with your clients.

RECOMMENDED READINGS

Association for Specialists in Group Work. (1989). *Ethical guidelines for group counselors.* Alexandria, VA: Author. These updated and expanded guidelines provide an adequate framework for group leaders to develop a professional orientation to their practice of group work. The guidelines appear in their entirety in Appendix A.

Atkinson, D. R., Morten, G., & Sue, D. W. (1993). *Counseling American minorities* (4th ed.). Madison, WI: Brown & Benchmark. The authors describe a minority-identity development model. This edited book has excellent sections dealing with counseling for Native Americans, Asian Americans, Blacks, and Latinos. It helps those who lead groups develop an awareness of cultural issues that affect the members' willingness to take part in group exercises and activities.

Blatner, A. (1988). *Acting-in: Practical applications of psychodramatic methods* (2nd ed.). New York: Springer. This excellent book describes the basic elements of psychodrama. Blatner describes techniques such as the auxiliary ego, the double, the warm-up, and approaches leading to action. He also focuses on training in the use of these methods.

Blatner, A., with Blatner, A. (1988). *Foundations of psychodrama: History, theory, and practice* (3rd ed.). New York: Springer. This is an excellent resource that deals with the historical, philosophical, psychological, social, and practical foundations of psychodrama. The authors have a readable style, and they present a fine overview of the practical applications of psychodrama.

Burnside, I. M. (Ed.). (1984). *Working with the elderly: Group process and techniques* (2nd ed.). Boston: Jones & Bartlett. This compendium contains a wealth of practical information and hints on subjects such as training and supervision, group membership issues and procedures, special types of groups for the elderly, guidelines for group workers, and the future of group work with the aged.

Carroll, M., & Wiggins, J. (1990). *Elements of group counseling: Back to the basics.* Denver: Love. This practical new book covers leadership roles, expectations of group members, and group leadership skills. It provides a variety of intervention techniques that are useful in peer support groups, single-parent groups, substance-abuse groups, AIDS groups, and school groups.

Corey, G. (1995). *Theory and practice of group counseling* (4th ed.). Pacific Grove, CA: Brooks/Cole. This text surveys the key concepts and techniques that flow from the major theories of group counseling. It also discusses the stages of groups, group membership, group leadership, and ethical and professional issues in group practice. A student manual with exercises and techniques for small groups is also available.

Corey, G. (1996a). *Case approach to counseling and psychotherapy* (4th ed.). Pacific Grove, CA: Brooks/Cole. This book presents separate case studies along with ideas for techniques drawn from contemporary counseling approaches. Experts from each of the various orientations demonstrate their respective approaches and styles in working with the same client. The techniques described are also applicable to working with clients in groups.

Corey, G. (1996b). *Theory and practice of counseling and psychotherapy* (5th ed.). Pacific Grove, CA: Brooks/Cole. This book describes nine therapeutic models that are applicable to both individual and group therapy. It also discusses basic issues in counseling, ethical issues, and the counselor as a person. The book is designed to give the reader an overview of the theoretical bases of the practice of counseling. A student manual is available to assist readers in applying the concepts to their personal growth.

Corey, G., & Corey, M. (1997). *I never knew I had a choice* (6th ed.). Pacific Grove, CA: Brooks/Cole. This book reviews many existential concerns and issues that clients bring to therapy such as those dealing with themes of childhood and adolescence, the struggle toward autonomy, work and leisure, the body and stress management, work, love, sex, sex roles, intimacy, loneliness, death, and meaning. The book discusses the bases on which we make choices for ourselves and how we shape our lives by the choices we make. It contains many exercises and activities that leaders can use for their group work and that they can suggest as homework assignments between sessions. Each chapter is followed by numerous annotated suggestions for further reading.

Corey, G., Corey, M. S., & Callanan, P. J. (1993). *Issues and ethics in the helping professions* (4th ed.). Pacific Grove, CA: Brooks/Cole. A combination of textbook and student manual, this book contains self-inventories, open-ended cases, exercises, and suggested activities. It deals with a range of professional issues pertinent to group work.

Corey, M. S., & Corey, G. (1993). *Becoming a helper* (2nd ed.). Pacific Grove, CA: Brooks/Cole. This book deals with the personal and professional lives of helpers. A few of the topics that have special relevance to group counselors include the motivations for becoming helpers, value issues, common concerns facing counselors, managing stress, dealing with professional burnout, and ethical issues in practice.

Corey, M. S., & Corey, G. (1997). *Groups: Process and practice* (5th ed.). Pacific Grove, CA: Brooks/Cole. Part One deals with the basic issues in group work. In Part Two separate chapters deal with group-process issues at each phase in the evolution of a group. Part Three describes specific types of groups for children, adolescents, adults, and the elderly.

Dies, R. R., & MacKenzie, K. R. (Eds.). (1983). *Advances in group psychotherapy: Integrating research and practice.* New York: International Universities Press. This book is aimed at bridging the gap between research and practice in group therapy. Dies stresses the role of the therapist as a model-setting participant and technical expert who provides a therapeutic structure in which meaningful interactions can occur.

Dinkmeyer, D. C., Dinkmeyer, D. C., Jr., & Sperry, L. (1987). *Adlerian counseling and psychotherapy* (2nd ed.). Columbus, OH: Merrill. This book is a clear and readable source with ideas for working with children, adults, adolescents, and families in groups. It contains concise descriptions of Adlerian techniques that can be used in groups.

Donigian, J., & Malnati, R. (1987). *Critical incidents in group therapy.* Pacific Grove, CA: Brooks/Cole. The aim of this book is to provide a theoretical rationale that will guide practitioners in working with a variety of groups. The core of the book consists of six leading practitioners responding to six typical critical points in the development of a group.

Duncan, J. A., & Gumaer, J. (Eds.). (1980). *Developmental groups for children.* Springfield, IL: Charles C Thomas. Contains several chapters on counseling children in groups. Other chapters deal with play therapy, art therapy, music therapy, bibliotherapy, behavioral counseling, and relaxation approaches.

Feder, B., & Ronall, R. (Eds.). (1980). *Beyond the hot seat: Gestalt approaches to group.* New York: Brunner/Mazel. This book contains some informative articles on the process of Gestalt groups along with techniques to use with various populations. It includes descriptions of art therapy in groups, movement therapy in groups, and marathons.

Friedman, W. H. (1989). *Practical group therapy.* San Francisco: Jossey-Bass. In this guide for clinicians, the author has separate chapters on topics such as techniques to enhance therapeutic factors in group work, coping with difficult members, special issues in group therapy, techniques for termination, role-playing techniques, and working with dreams.

Gazda, G. (Ed.). (1981). *Innovations to group psychotherapy* (2nd ed.). Springfield, IL: Charles C Thomas. Some chapters include multiple-impact training (groups for training in life skills), logotherapy groups, the person-centered approach applied to large groups, rational behavior therapy in groups, and theme-centered interactional therapy.

Gazda, G. (1989). *Group counseling: A developmental approach* (4th ed.). Boston: Allyn & Bacon. This is a basic book on group counseling. It contains chapters on group procedures for preschoolers, young children, preadolescents, adolescents, and adults. It also covers group counseling research and ethical and professional issues.

Glasser, W. (1985). *Control theory.* New York: Harper & Row (Perennial Paperback). Contains the most recent updating of reality therapy. It is a nontechnical book that illustrates ways of using control theory to deal with relationship problems, alcoholism, depression, diseases, child-rearing questions, and weight problems. Glasser's philosophy can easily be incorporated into the structure of a group.

Jacobs, E. E., Harvill, R. L., Masson, R. L. (1994). *Group counseling: Strategies and skills* (2nd ed.). Pacific Grove, CA: Brooks/Cole. The authors have specific chapters on the topics of dealing with problem situations and working with specific populations, as well as other general chapters on group process. They have several chapters dealing with skills of cutting off and drawing out, making the rounds, and the use of exercises. One of their chapters is devoted to introducing, conducting, and processing exercises.

Johnson, D. W. (1990). *Reaching out: Interpersonal effectiveness and self-actualization* (4th ed.). Englewood Cliffs, NJ: Prentice-Hall. Designed to provide the theory and experience necessary to develop effective interpersonal skills, this book provides many exercises that can be applied in a group setting. Some topics include self-disclosure, developing and maintaining trust, expressing feelings verbally and nonverbally, listening and responding, resolving interpersonal conflicts, managing anger and stress, and barriers to interpersonal effectiveness.

Johnson, D. W., & Johnson, F. P. (1991). *Joining together: Group theory and group skills* (4th ed.). Englewood Cliffs, NJ: Prentice-Hall. Reviews current social psychological knowledge on small groups and provides a wide range of group exercises to build skills in effective group membership and leadership. Some topics include group dynamics leadership, decision making, communication within groups, conflicts of interests, use of power, leading growth and counseling groups, team building, psychological benefits of group membership.

Kaplan, H. I., & Sadock, B. J. (Eds.). (1983). *Comprehensive group psychotherapy* (2nd ed.). Baltimore: Williams & Wilkins. This is a useful reference work. It covers a wide range of topics such as basic principles of groups, specialized group-therapy techniques, approaches to group therapy, groups with specialized populations, issues in training and research, and groups in the international scene.

Kottler, J. A. (1993). *On being a therapist* (Rev. ed.). San Francisco: Jossey-Bass. This book focuses on how therapists' work directly affects their personal life. By becoming involved in the exploration of their clients' pain, therapists also become open to their own psychological wounds. The author gives examples of the price that therapists pay for this stressful profession. Group counselors can benefit personally by reviewing and reflecting on the themes in this work.

Kottler, J. A. (1994). *Advanced group leadership*. Pacific Grove, CA: Brooks/Cole. An appropriate book for a course that describes how people change in groups and the dimensions of group leadership. Kottler also has chapters describing group-leadership strategies such as risk taking, creative metaphors, the use of humor, and adjunct structures. The final chapter deals with common unethical behaviors in groups.

Kottler, J. A. (1991). *The compleat therapist*. San Francisco: Jossey-Bass. This book examines the variables that are common to most therapies, deals with what therapists do with clients that makes a difference, and addresses the personal factors that enhance therapeutic effectiveness. Although this book is not on group techniques, much of the content could be usefully applied to group practice.

Kottler, J. A., & Blau, D. S. (1989). *The imperfect therapist: Learning from failure in therapeutic practice*. San Francisco: Jossey-Bass. The authors describe how unrealistic expectations and perfectionism can influence therapists' experience of failure. They write about the common mistakes of beginning therapists and show how they can learn from these experiences. The content covered in this book has much relevance for group leaders who burden themselves with perfectionistic standards.

Lakin, M. (1985). *The helping group: Therapeutic principles and issues*. Reading, MA: Addison-Wesley. The author has a particularly useful chapter on ethical issues in helping groups. There is also a separate chapter on the nature and purpose of self-help groups.

Leveton, E. (1977). *Psychodrama for the timid clinician*. New York: Springer. The author offers an excellent view of psychodramatic techniques. Group leaders can benefit greatly from reading the book and following the author's advice to use experimental techniques in group work.

Luft, J. (1984). *Group processes: An introduction to group dynamics* (3rd ed.). Palo Alto, CA: Mayfield. Explores the basic issues fundamental to groups, such as leadership, communication, group effectiveness, and conflict. Part One deals with group processes in perspective, with a focus on stages of group development. Part Two deals with models and metaphors. Featured in this section are discussions of the Johari window, the Zucchini connection, and Bales's interaction-process analysis. Part Three is concerned with the interpersonal influences in groups. Part Four describes specific techniques and applications.

Morganett, R. S. (1990). *Skills for living: Group counseling activities for young adolescents*. Champaign, IL: Research Press. This is a very useful handbook for practitioners who work with children and adolescents. The author presents exercises and techniques that can be used in the following types of groups: dealing with divorce; making and keeping friends; learning communication and assertion skills; developing self-esteem; acquiring stress-management skills; acquiring anger-management skills; school survival and success; and coping with grief and loss.

Napier, R. W., & Gershenfeld, M. K. (1983). *Making groups work: A guide for group leaders.* Boston: Houghton Mifflin. Explores issues of why some groups fail and some groups succeed. Specific chapters deal with the group leader's role, questions asked by leaders, designs for groups, interventions for conflict situations, and evaluation.

Napier, R. W., & Gershenfeld, M. K. (1989). *Groups: Theory and experience* (4th ed.). Boston: Houghton Mifflin. A group-dynamics text that deals with a range of topics, including group norms, membership and leadership issues, goals, group problem solving and decision making, the evolution of groups, and the use of humor in small groups.

Nicholas, M. W. (1984). *Change in the context of group therapy.* New York: Brunner/Mazel. Deals with how individuals' frames of reference are changing in group. Shows how members change their perspectives by adopting new roles and by reframing of their own experience through experimentation and feedback in a group.

Oaklander, V. (1978). *Windows to our children. A Gestalt approach to children and adolescents.* Moab, UT: Real People Press. This is a how-to book that describes the author's work with children in a very sensitive and straightforward manner. Many of her techniques can be applied to young people in group settings.

Ohlsen, M. M., Horne, A. M., & Lawe, C. F. (1988). *Group counseling* (3rd ed.). New York: Holt, Rinehart & Winston. The authors have useful ideas for leaders who want to work with structured groups. They also have several chapters on working with resistance and learning to challenge reluctant clients.

Peck, M. S. (1987). *The different drum: Community making and peace.* The author deals with the true meaning of community, the genesis of community, and the stages of community-making, all of which seem to apply to our weeklong residential workshops and the techniques that we have developed.

Pedersen, P. (1994). *A handbook for developing multicultural awareness* (2nd ed.). Alexandria, VA: American Counseling Association. The material in this book will be most helpful for group counselors who are interested in expanding their awareness of a multicultural perspective in group work. The author makes the assumption that all counseling is to some extent multicultural, and he maintains that we can either choose to attend to the influence of culture or ignore it. This useful handbook deals with topics such as becoming aware of our culturally biased assumptions, acquiring knowledge for effective multicultural counseling, and learning skills to deal with cultural diversity.

Perls, F. (1969). *Gestalt therapy verbatim.* Moab, UT: Real People Press. Perls gives an informal, easy-to-read description of most of the basic concepts of Gestalt therapy. Of particular interest are discussions of the goals of therapy, responsibility, the client/therapist relationship, diagnosis, and the functions and roles of the therapist.

Powers, R. L., & Griffith, J. (1987). *Understanding life-style: The psycho-clarity process.* Chicago: The Americas Institute of Adlerian Studies. Many clinical examples make this book useful. Separate chapters deal with interview techniques, lifestyle assessment, early recollections, the family constellation, and methods of summarizing and interpreting information.

Rainwater, J. (1979). *You're in charge: A guide to becoming your own therapist.* Los Angeles: Guild of Tutors Press. This excellent self-help book provides leaders with ideas for using journals, autobiographies, and fantasy approaches in groups.

Rogers, C. (1970). *Carl Rogers on encounter groups.* New York: Harper & Row. This readable book on the process of the basic encounter group deals with how leaders can be facilitative and what changes occur in people and in organizations as a result of participating in encounter groups.

Rose, S. D. (1989). *Working with adults in groups.* San Francisco: Jossey-Bass. This is an excellent book from a behavioral orientation that deals with starting and conducting groups, using behavioral strategies, and developing techniques for helping members extend therapy into the real world. Many specific techniques are outlined.

Rose, S. D., & Edleson, J. L. (1987). *Working with children and adolescents in groups: A multimethod approach.* San Francisco: Jossey-Bass. Separate chapters deal with orienting group members, assessing problems of members, and techniques for changing behavior in groups. Specific techniques are described that will be useful for those who work in groups with children and adolescents.

Shaffer, J., & Galinsky, M. D. (1989). *Models of group therapy* (2nd ed.). Englewood Cliffs, NJ: Prentice-Hall. This book deals with some of the various models of group therapy, such as psychodrama, Gestalt therapy, and behavior therapy. There are also separate chapters on different types of groups such as the encounter group, the self-help group, the theme-centered group, and the laboratory group. Each of these groups have special techniques.

Sue, D. W., & Sue, D. (1990). *Counseling the culturally different: Theory and practice* (2nd ed.). New York: Wiley. This book is based on the assumption that cultural diversity is a fact of life and that therapeutic practice should reflect an understanding of this diversity. A careful reading will help group counselors adapt their techniques to the cultural background of the members. The authors show how traditional counseling approaches may clash with cultural values, and they suggest alternative ways of dealing with the critical incidents that often occur in therapy.

Vander Kolk, C. J. (1990). *Introduction to group counseling and psychotherapy.* Prospect Heights, IL: Waveland Press. This book provides an overview of models of group counseling and deals with issues in group practice. The author covers group work with special populations such as the disabled, children and adolescents, families, and couples.

Wubbolding, R. E. (1988). *Using reality therapy.* New York: Harper & Row (Perennial Library). This book is clearly written, with many practical guidelines for using the principles of reality therapy in practice. It covers a range of techniques that can be applied to group work. The author describes strategies such as paradoxical intention, the use of humor, creating action plans, the skillful use of questions, self-help techniques, and ways of challenging clients to look at what they are doing.

Yalom, I. D. (1980). *Existential psychotherapy.* New York: Basic Books. This book provides an outstanding foundation for group counselors who are interested in dealing with universal human themes. Substantial chapters deal with the themes of death, freedom, isolation, and meaninglessness.

Yalom, I. D. (1983). *Inpatient group psychotherapy.* New York: Basic Books. Highly readable book for group therapists who work with both higher- and lower-level inpatient groups. The focus is on general principles of therapy and strategies and techniques of leadership. Techniques are given for a single-session time frame and also for short-term groups with a here-and-now focus.

Yalom, I. D. (1995). *The theory and practice of group psychotherapy* (4th ed.). New York: Basic Books. An excellent and comprehensive text on group therapy, this book presents detailed discussions of the therapeutic factors in groups, the group therapist, issues of transference and transparency, procedures in organizing therapy groups, problem patients, techniques with specialized formats and procedural aids, specialized therapy groups, group therapy compared with the encounter group, and the training of group therapists.

Zimpfer, D. G. (1984). *Group work in the helping professions: A bibliography.* Muncie, IN: Accelerated Development. A comprehensive source of articles and books dealing with a panorama of group issues such as understanding group dynamics and processes, planning and implementation of groups, types of group experience or approach, groups with specific populations, outcome studies, group and individual treatments, new directions, ethical and professional issues in groups, and training and supervision of group workers.

Zinker, J. (1978). *Creative process in Gestalt therapy.* New York: Random House (Vintage). A beautifully written book that captures the essence of Gestalt therapy. The author shows how the therapist functions much like an artist in creating experiments that encourage clients to expand their boundaries. This work shows the difference between planned exercises that are imposed on clients and experiments that grow out of the therapeutic process.

Ethical Guidelines for Group Counselors
ASGW 1989 Revision

Association for Specialists in Group Work

PREAMBLE

One characteristic of any professional group is the possession of a body of knowledge, skills, and voluntarily, self-professed standards for ethical practice. A Code of Ethics consists of those standards that have been formally and publicly acknowledged by the members of a profession to serve as the guidelines for professional conduct, discharge of duties, and the resolution of moral dilemmas. By this document, the Association for Specialists in Group Work (ASGW) has identified the standards of conduct appropriate for ethical behavior among its members.

The Association for Specialists in Group Work recognizes the basic commitment of its members to the Ethical Standards of its parent organization, the American Association for Counseling and Development (AACD) and nothing in this document shall be construed to supplant that code. These standards are intended to complement the AACD standards in the area of group work by clarifying the nature of ethical responsibility of the counselor in the group setting and by stimulating a greater concern for competent group leadership.

The group counselor is expected to be a professional agent and to take the processes of ethical responsibility seriously. ASGW views "ethical process" as being integral to group work and views group counselors as "ethical agents." Group counselors, by their very nature in being responsible and responsive to their group members, necessarily embrace a certain potential for ethical vulnerability. It is incumbent upon group counselors to give considerable attention to the intent and context of their actions because the attempts of counselors to influence human behavior through group work always have ethical implications.

The following ethical guidelines have been developed to encourage ethical behavior of group counselors. These guidelines are written for students and practitioners, and are meant to stimulate reflection, self-examination, and discussion of issues and practices. They address the group counselor's responsibility for providing information about group work to clients and the group counselor's responsibility for providing group counseling services to clients. A final section discusses the group counselor's responsibility for safeguarding ethical practice and procedures for reporting unethical behavior. Group counselors are expected to make known these standards to group members.

ETHICAL GUIDELINES

1. *Orientation and Providing Information:* Group counselors adequately prepare prospective or new group members by providing as much information about the existing or proposed group as necessary.
   - Minimally, information related to each of the following areas should be provided.
     a. Entrance procedures, time parameters of the group experience, group participation expec-

From *ASGW Ethical Guidelines for Group Counselors*, Volume 15, Number 2, May 1990, 119–126. © American Association for Counseling and Development. Reprinted with permission. These guidelines were approved by the Association for Specialists in Group Work (ASGW) Executive Board, June 1, 1989.

tations, methods of payment (where appropriate), and termination procedures are explained by the group counselor as appropriate to the level of maturity of group members and the nature and purpose(s) of the group.

b. Group counselors have available for distribution, a professional disclosure statement that includes information on the group counselor's qualifications and group services that can be provided, particularly as related to the nature and purpose(s) of the specific group.

c. Group counselors communicate the role expectations, rights, and responsibilities of group members and group counselor(s).

d. The group goals are stated as concisely as possible by the group counselor including "whose" goal it is (the group counselor's, the institution's, the parent's, the law's, society's, etc.) and the role of group members in influencing or determining the group's goal(s).

e. Group counselors explore with group members the risks of potential life changes that may occur because of the group experience and help members explore their readiness to face these possibilities.

f. Group members are informed by the group counselor of unusual or experimental procedures that might be expected in their group experience.

g. Group counselors explain, as realistically as possible, what services can and cannot be provided within the particular group structure offered.

h. Group counselors emphasize the need to promote full psychological functioning and presence among group members. They inquire from prospective group members whether they are using any kind of drug or medication that may affect functioning in the group. They do not permit any use of alcohol and/or illegal drugs during group sessions and they discourage the use of alcohol and/or drugs (legal or illegal) prior to group meetings which may affect the physical or emotional presence of the member or other group members.

i. Group counselors inquire from prospective group members whether they have ever been a client in counseling or psychotherapy. If a prospective group member is already in a counseling relationship with another professional person, the group counselor advises the prospective group member to notify the other professional of their participation in the group.

j. Group counselors clearly inform group members about the policies pertaining to the group counselor's willingness to consult with them between group sessions.

k. In establishing fees for group counseling services, group counselors consider the financial status and the locality of prospective group members. Group members are not charged fees for group sessions where the group counselor is not present and the policy of charging for sessions missed by a group member is clearly communicated. Fees for participating as a group member are contracted between group counselor and group member for a specified period of time. Group counselors do not increase fees for group counseling services until the existing contracted fee structure has expired. In the event that the established fee structure is inappropriate for a prospective member, group counselors assist in finding comparable services of acceptable cost.

2. *Screening of Members:* The group counselor screens prospective group members (when appropriate to their

theoretical orientation). Insofar as possible, the counselor selects group members whose needs and goals are compatible with the goals of the group, who will not impede the group process, and whose well-being will not be jeopardized by the group experience. An orientation to the group (i.e., ASGW Ethical Guideline #1), is included during the screening process.

- Screening may be accomplished in one or more ways, such as the following:
  a. Individual interview,
  b. Group interview of prospective group members,
  c. Interview as part of a team staffing, and,
  d. Completion of a written questionnaire by prospective group members.

3. *Confidentiality:* Group counselors protect members by defining clearly what confidentiality means, why it is important, and the difficulties involved in enforcement.

   a. Group counselors take steps to protect members by defining confidentiality and the limits of confidentiality (i.e., when a group member's condition indicates that there is clear and imminent danger to the member, others, or physical property, the group counselor takes reasonable personal action and/or informs responsible authorities).

   b. Group counselors stress the importance of confidentiality and set a norm of confidentiality regarding all group participants' disclosures. The importance of maintaining confidentiality is emphasized before the group begins and at various times in the group. The fact that confidentiality cannot be guaranteed is clearly stated.

   c. Members are made aware of the difficulties involved in enforcing and ensuring confidentiality in a group setting. The counselor provides examples of how confidentiality can non-maliciously be broken to increase members' awareness, and help to lessen the likelihood that this breach of confidence will occur. Group counselors inform group members about the potential consequences of intentionally breaching confidentiality.

   d. Group counselors can only ensure confidentiality on their part and not on the part of the members.

   e. Group counselors video or audio tape a group session only with the prior consent, and the members' knowledge of how the tape will be used.

   f. When working with minors, the group counselor specifies the limits of confidentiality.

   g. Participants in a mandatory group are made aware of any reporting procedures required of the group counselor.

   h. Group counselors store or dispose of group member records (written, audio, video, etc.) in ways that maintain confidentiality.

   i. Instructors of group counseling courses maintain the anonymity of group members whenever discussing group counseling cases.

4. *Voluntary/Involuntary Participation:* Group counselors inform members whether participation is voluntary or involuntary.

   a. Group counselors take steps to ensure informed consent procedures in both voluntary and involuntary groups.

   b. When working with minors in a group, counselors are expected to follow the procedures specified by the institution in which they are practicing.

   c. Within voluntary groups, every attempt is made to enlist the cooperation of the members and their continuance in the group on a voluntary basis.

   d. Group counselors do not certify that group treatment has been received by members who merely attend sessions, but did not meet the defined groups expectations. Group members are informed about the consequences for failing to participate in a group.

5. *Leaving a Group:* Provisions are made to assist a group member to terminate in an effective way.
   a. Procedures to be followed for a group member who chooses to exit a group prematurely are discussed by the counselor with all group members either before the group begins, during a pre-screening interview, or during the initial group session.
   b. In the case of legally mandated group counseling, group counselors inform members of the possible consequences for premature self-termination.
   c. Ideally, both the group counselor and the member can work cooperatively to determine the degree to which a group experience is productive or counterproductive for that individual.
   d. Members ultimately have a right to discontinue membership in the group, at a designated time, if the predetermined trial period proves to be unsatisfactory.
   e. Members have the right to exit a group, but it is important that they be made aware of the importance of informing the counselor and the group members prior to deciding to leave. The counselor discusses the possible risks of leaving the group prematurely with a member who is considering this option.
   f. Before leaving a group, the group counselor encourages members (if appropriate) to discuss their reasons for wanting to discontinue membership in the group. Counselors intervene if other members use undue pressure to force a member to remain in the group.
6. *Coercion and Pressure:* Group counselors protect member rights against physical threats, intimidation, coercion, and undue peer pressure insofar as is reasonably possible.
   a. It is essential to differentiate between "therapeutic pressure" that is part of any group and "undue pressure," which is not therapeutic.

b. The purpose of a group is to help participants find their own answer, not to pressure them into doing what the group thinks is appropriate.
c. Counselors exert care not to coerce participants to change in directions which they clearly state they do not choose.
d. Counselors have a responsibility to intervene when others use undue pressure or attempt to persuade members against their will.
e. Counselors intervene when any member attempts to act out aggression in a physical way that might harm another member or themselves.
f. Counselors intervene when a member is verbally abusive or inappropriately confrontive to another member.

7. *Imposing Counselor Values:* Group counselors develop an awareness of their own values and needs and the potential impact they have on the interventions likely to be made.
   a. Although group counselors take care to avoid imposing their values on members, it is appropriate that they expose their own beliefs, decisions, needs, and values, when concealing them would create problems for the members.
   b. There are values implicit in any group, and these are made clear to potential members before they join the group. (Examples of certain values include: expressing feelings, being direct and honest, sharing personal material with others, learning how to trust, improving interpersonal communication, and deciding for oneself.)
   c. Personal and professional needs of group counselors are not met at the members' expense.
   d. Group counselors avoid using the group for their own therapy.
   e. Group counselors are aware of their own values and assumptions and how these apply in a multicultural context.
   f. Group counselors take steps to in-

crease their awareness of ways that their personal reactions to members might inhibit the group process and they monitor their countertransference. Through an awareness of the impact of stereotyping and discrimination (i.e., biases based on age, disability, ethnicity, gender, race, religion, or sexual preference), group counselors guard the individual rights and personal dignity of all group members.

8. *Equitable Treatment:* Group counselors make every reasonable effort to treat each member individually and equally.

   a. Group counselors recognize and respect differences (e.g., cultural, racial, religious, lifestyle, age, disability, gender) among group members.

   b. Group counselors maintain an awareness of their behavior toward individual group members and are alert to the potential detrimental effects of favoritism or partiality toward any particular group member to the exclusion or detriment of any other member(s). It is likely that group counselors will favor some members over others, yet all group members deserve to be treated equally.

   c. Group counselors ensure equitable use of group time for each member by inviting silent members to become involved, acknowledging nonverbal attempts to communicate, and discouraging rambling and monopolizing of time by members.

   d. If a large group is planned, counselors consider enlisting another qualified professional to serve as a co-leader for the group sessions.

9. *Dual Relationships:* Group counselors avoid dual relationships with group members that might impair their objectivity and professional judgment, as well as those which are likely to compromise a group member's ability to participate fully in the group.

   a. Group counselors do not misuse their professional role and power as group leader to advance personal or social contacts with members throughout the duration of the group.

   b. Group counselors do not use their professional relationship with group members to further their own interest either during the group or after the termination of the group.

   c. Sexual intimacies between group counselors and members are unethical.

   d. Group counselors do not barter (exchange) professional services with group members for services.

   e. Group counselors do not admit their own family members, relatives, employees, or personal friends as members to their groups.

   f. Group counselors discuss with group members the potential detrimental effects of group members engaging in intimate intermember relationships outside of the group.

   g. Students who participate in a group as a partial course requirement for a group course are not evaluated for an academic grade based upon their degree of participation as a member in a group. Instructors of group counseling courses take steps to minimize the possible negative impact on students when they participate in a group course by separating course grades from participation in the group and by allowing students to decide what issues to explore and when to stop.

   h. It is inappropriate to solicit members from a class (or institutional affiliation) for one's private counseling or therapeutic groups.

10. *Use of Techniques:* Group counselors do not attempt any technique unless trained in its use or under supervision by a counselor familiar with the intervention.

    a. Group counselors are able to

articulate a theoretical orientation that guides their practice, and they are able to provide a rationale for their interventions.

b. Depending upon the type of an intervention, group counselors have training commensurate with the potential impact of a technique.

c. Group counselors are aware of the necessity to modify their techniques to fit the unique needs of various cultural and ethnic groups.

d. Group counselors assist members in translating in-group learnings to daily life.

11. *Goal Development:* Group counselors make every effort to assist members in developing their personal goals.

a. Group counselors use their skills to assist members in making their goals specific so that others present in the group will understand the nature of the goals.

b. Throughout the course of a group, group counselors assist members in assessing the degree to which personal goals are being met, and assist in revising any goals when it is appropriate.

c. Group counselors help members clarify the degree to which the goals can be met within the context of a particular group.

12. *Consultation:* Group counselors develop and explain policies about between-session consultation to group members.

a. Group counselors take care to make certain that members do not use between-session consultations to avoid dealing with issues pertaining to the group that would be dealt with best in the group.

b. Group counselors urge members to bring the issues discussed during between-session consultations into the group if they pertain to the group.

c. Group counselors seek out consultation and/or supervision regarding ethical concerns or when encountering difficulties which interfere with their effective functioning as group leaders.

d. Group counselors seek appropriate professional assistance for their own personal problems or conflicts that are likely to impair their professional judgment and work performance.

e. Group counselors discuss their group cases only for professional consultation and educational purposes.

f. Group counselors inform members about policies regarding whether consultation will be held confidential.

13. *Termination from the Group:* Depending upon the purpose of participation in the group, counselors promote termination of members from the group in the most efficient period of time.

a. Group counselors maintain a constant awareness of the progress made by each group member and periodically invite the group members to explore and reevaluate their experiences in the group. It is the responsibility of group counselors to help promote the independence of members from the group in a timely manner.

14. *Evaluation and Follow-up:* Group counselors make every attempt to engage in ongoing assessment and to design follow-up procedures for their groups.

a. Group counselors recognize the importance of ongoing assessment of a group, and they assist members in evaluating their own progress.

b. Group counselors conduct evaluation of the total group experience at the final meeting (or before termination), as well as ongoing evaluation.

c. Group counselors monitor their own behavior and become aware of what they are modeling in the group.

d. Follow-up procedures might take the form of personal contact, telephone contact, or written contact.

e. Follow-up meetings might be with individuals, or groups, or both to determine the degree to which: (i) members have reached their goals, (ii) the group had a positive or negative effect on the participants, (iii) members could profit from some type of referral, and (iv) as information for possible modification of future groups. If there is no follow-up meeting, provisions are made available for individual follow-up meetings to any member who needs or requests such a contact.

15. *Referrals:* If the needs of a particular member cannot be met within the type of group being offered, the group counselor suggests other appropriate professional referrals.
    a. Group counselors are knowledgeable of local community resources for assisting group members regarding professional referrals.
    b. Group counselors help members seek further professional assistance, if needed.

16. *Professional Development:* Group counselors recognize that professional growth is a continuous, ongoing, developmental process throughout their career.
    a. Group counselors maintain and upgrade their knowledge and skill competencies through educational activities, clinical experiences, and participation in professional development activities.
    b. Group counselors keep abreast of research findings and new developments as applied to groups.

SAFEGUARDING ETHICAL PRACTICE AND PROCEDURES FOR REPORTING UNETHICAL BEHAVIOR

The preceding remarks have been advanced as guidelines which are generally representative of ethical and professional group practice. They have not been proposed as rigidly defined prescriptions. However, practitioners who are thought to be grossly unresponsive to the ethical concerns addressed in this document may be subject to a review of their practices by the AACD Ethics Committee and ASGW peers.

• For consultation and/or questions regarding these ASGW Ethical Guidelines or group ethical dilemmas, you may contact the Chairperson of the ASGW Ethics Committee. The name, address, and telephone number of the current ASGW Ethics Committee Chairperson may be acquired by telephoning the AACD office in Alexandria Virginia at (703) 823-9800.

• If a group counselor's behavior is suspected as being unethical, the following procedures are to be followed:
    a. Collect more information and investigate further to confirm the unethical practice as determined by the ASGW Ethical Guidelines.
    b. Confront the individual with the apparent violation of ethical guidelines for the purposes of protecting the safety of any clients and to help the group counselor correct any inappropriate behaviors. If satisfactory resolution is not reached through this contact then:
    c. A complaint should be made in writing, including the specific facts and dates of the alleged violation and all relevant supporting data. The complaint should be included in an envelope marked "CONFIDENTIAL" to ensure confidentiality for both the accuser(s) and the alleged violator(s) and forwarded to all of the following sources:

1. The name and address of the Chairperson of the state Counselor Licensure Board for the respective state, if in existence.
2. The Ethics Committee
   c/o The President
   American Association for
       Counseling
       and Development
   5999 Stevenson Avenue
   Alexandria, Virginia 22304
3. The name and address of all private credentialing agencies that the alleged violator maintains credentials or holds professional membership. Some of these include the following:

National Board for Certified
Counselors, Inc.
5999 Stevenson Avenue
Alexandria, Virginia 22304

National Council for Credentialing
of Career Counselors
c/o NBCC
5999 Stevenson Avenue
Alexandria, Virginia 22304

National Academy for Certified
Clinical Mental Health Counselors
5999 Stevenson Avenue
Alexandria, Virginia 22304

Commission on Rehabilitation
Counselor Certification
162 North State Street, Suite 317
Chicago, Illinois 60601

American Association for Marriage
and Family Therapy
1717 K Street, N. W., Suite 407
Washington, D.C. 20006

American Psychological Association
1200 Seventeenth Street, N.W.
Washington, D.C. 20036

American Group Psychotherapy
Association, Inc.
25 East 21st Street, 6th Floor
New York, New York 10010

Information on Professional Organizations for Group Workers

For information about joining the ASGW, contact the address given below. Members receive the *Journal for Specialists in Group Work*, which is published in March, May, September, and November. The journal is an excellent source for staying current in the field in the areas of research, working with groups, innovations and ideas, and reviews and developments.

American Association for
Counseling and Development
5999 Stevenson Avenue
Alexandria, VA 22304
(703) 823-9800

Another source for keeping current in group therapy is the *International Journal of Group Psychotherapy*, which is published in January, April, July, and October. It is published by the American Group Psychotherapy Association, which is another excellent professional organization to belong to if you are interested in group therapy. The membership fee for the AGPA includes the subscription to the above journal. For information contact:

American Group Psychotherapy
Association
25 East 21st Street, 6th Floor
New York, NY 10010

INDEX

To the owner of this book:

We enjoyed writing *Group Techniques*, and it is our hope that you have enjoyed reading it. We'd like to know about your experiences with the book; only through your comments and the comments of others can we assess the impact of this book and make it better.

School: _____

Instructor's name: _____

1. What did you like *most* about the book? _____

_____

_____

_____

2. What did you like *least* about the book? _____

_____

_____

_____

3. How useful were the *questions and activities* at the end of the chapters? _____

_____

_____

4. What class did you use this book for? _____

_____

5. In the space below or in a separate letter, please tell us what it was like for you to read this book and how you used it. Please give your suggestions for revisions and any other comments you'd like to make about the book. Include, if you'd like, your own ideas for group techniques.

Optional:

Your name: _____ Date: _____

May Brooks/Cole quote you, either in promotion for *Group Techniques*, Second Edition, or in future publishing ventures?

Yes _____ No _____

Sincerely,

Gerald Corey
Marianne Schneider Corey
Patrick J. Callanan
J. Michael Russell

FOLD HERE

NO POSTAGE
NECESSARY
IF MAILED
IN THE
UNITED STATES

BUSINESS REPLY MAIL
FIRST CLASS   PERMIT NO. 358   PACIFIC GROVE, CA

POSTAGE WILL BE PAID BY ADDRESSEE

ATT: Corey, Corey, Callanan, Russell
_____

Brooks/Cole Publishing Company
511 Forest Lodge Road
Pacific Grove, California 93950-9968

FOLD HERE